Guides to Youth Ministry

PASTORAL CARE

Edited by
SHARON REED

THE WORLD OF
DON BOSCO
MULTIMEDIA

New Rochelle, NY

Guides to Youth Ministry: Pastoral Care

is published as a service for adults who love the young and want to share the Gospel with them.

It is a guide to understanding the young and a resource book for helping them. As such, it is addressed to parish, parish youth ministers, clergy who work with the young, and teachers.

Other *Guides to Youth Ministry* available:

Retreats

EarlyAdolescent Ministry

Spirituality

Justice

Evangelization

Liturgy and Worship

Media and Culture

Prepared in collaboration with
The Center for Youth Ministry Development

Guides to Youth Ministry: Pastoral Care
© 1993 Don Bosco Multimedia
475 North Avenue, P.O. Box T, New Rochelle, NY 10802
All rights reserved.

Library of Congress Cataloging-in-Publication Data
Pastoral Care/ edited by Sharon Reed.
p. cm.—(Guides to Youth Ministry)
Includes bibliographical references.
    1. Pastoral Care   2. Youth—Religious Life.
        I. Reed, Sharon   II. Pastoral Care   III. Series

ISBN 0-89944-268-4

Printed in the United States of America

9/93   9 8 7 6 5 4 3 2 1

CONTENTS

PART III: PRACTICAL APPROACHES FOR PASTORAL CARE

INTRODUCTION

In the foreword to *Clinical Handbook of Pastoral Counseling*, M. Scott Peck writes:

> We are, by God's grace, moving out of an age of excessive specialization into an age of integration. This profound movement from specialization to integration is both graceful and saving....because it is a movement toward integrity.... Integrity is never painless. It requires that we *do* let things rub against each other — that we fully experience life's conflicting demands and attempt to integrate them into resolutions of integrity.... The way of integrity is a way of tension.... The way of integrity is the way of the cross, and there is no other way to truth and healing (1-2).

Guides to Youth Ministry: Pastoral Care is an attempt to weave and integrate youth ministry and pastoral care so that one is almost unrecognizable without the other. A pastoral care approach appears repeatedly throughout the Scriptures, particularly in the Gospels, Paul's Letters, and Acts. Pastoral care approach has long been part of the foundation of parish ministry, particularly with individuals and families in crisis. Pastoral care has always been a part of the Church's mission and of the vision of outreach to young people.

Pastoral care has also had its own inherent tensions. In our efforts to avoid the tensions, we often took shortcuts. The shortcuts were often more efficient, but not necessarily more effective. In youth ministry, the shortcut was named "guidance and healing," one of the seven components listed in the original *A Vision of Youth Ministry*. Once we had pastoral care compartmentalized, it was taken care of — out of sight, out of mind. Each year as we evaluated our efforts in the arena of pastoral care, all we had to do was consult the heading "Guidance and Healing" and check it off. Completed. Finished. Achieved.

The *Guides to Youth Ministry: Pastoral Care* assumes that pastoral care is never fully achieved. It is a lens that provides a perspective on the process of youth ministry, not the outcome. Its emphasis is more relationship oriented rather than task oriented. It involves people "rubbing against each other" — parents, adolescents, youth ministers, teachers, pastors, community leaders — all trying to discover the best ways to integrate efforts and resources on behalf of healthy adolescent development. Sometimes the tension is incredible, but it is all part of the journey to integrity.

In *Raising Self-Reliant Children in a Self-Indulgent World*, Stephen Glenn and Jane Nelson state that "spiritual affirmation stems from self-affirmation" and that "three conditions are necessary for spiritual affirmation — to be listened to, to be taken seriously and to feel genuinely needed for one's own personal worth and contributions" (105). Pastoral care and youth ministry address these issues from different ends of the same spectrum — pastoral care provides the perspective and youth ministry the process. Now it is simply a matter of making both a priority! We simply need to reestablish the vision of who we are, what we stand for, and where we are headed. A pastoral care lens to youth ministry will show us *how* to get there!

Throughout the book you will discover several premises and principles that are emphasized again and again. The risks to healthy adolescent development have never been higher and the need for young people committed to spreading the kingdom message have never been more in demand. These principles are essential for us to understand what must be done and how to effectively serve as change agents. Take them to heart!

1. **Pastoral Care Is Not Counseling**. All youth ministers need to be pastoral caregivers; those who are professionally trained can also be counselors. There is an incredible difference. Pastoral care demands integrating sound theological principles with good interpersonal skills and programming. We are *not* advocating that youth ministers make interventions or diagnoses, or to hang out a shingle that says "counselor." Pastoral care requires strong self-knowledge, an understanding of the adolescent experience and family systems, and a caring stance toward the feelings of young people. Pastoral care provides support, guidance, confrontation when necessary, information, and tools for empowerment.

2. **Pastoral Care Is Not Limited to Crisis Situations**. This book contends that pastoral care is part of an ongoing relationship with individuals or groups. It is proactive rather than reactive. We are continually being challenged to look for new opportunities to care and to help teens and their parents negotiate the adolescent years as smoothly as possible. There will be developmental and situational crisis points that will demand a certain expertise, but an ongoing pastoral presence is also required.

3. **Pastoral Care Is A Community Responsibility.** Pastoral care moves beyond even parish and school boundaries to include local, diocesan, state, and even national attention. Young people are a very special resource. Many of them live in extremely at-risk situations, which include poverty, violence, lack of support systems, limited choices. Pastoral care must be a collaborative effort. Community networks must be established; resources shared; personnel skilled in dealing with adolescent issues targeted; and communication, programming, and advocacy addressed through a multi-faceted, comprehensive approach.

4. **Many Young People Lack the Life Skills Necessary to Prepare for the Future.** Because we have become so compartmentalized in our thinking, a gap has occurred in the skills taught to help adolescents cope and plan. We need to identify skills (intrapersonal, interpersonal, and systemic) essential to young people's survival and success. Models of competence must be made available. Developing the life skills of adolescents is an essential element of our pastoral care efforts.

5. **Pastoral Care Must Address the Needs of Families Experiencing Stress.** Family structures and family systems have changed tremendously in the twentieth century. Single-parent families and step-families abound. Parents are often not equipped to deal with their own identity issues, much less their children's. Teenagers often lose their place in the family structure at the very same time they are trying to identify where they belong in the larger scheme. The Church does not often provide a place for them either. Parents and adolescents need time and space in which to explore these issues in a caring environment with caring professionals.

As you can see from these five principles, this book proposes a broad understanding of pastoral care. Pastoral care includes three interdependent elements:

- promotion and prevention — strategies for promoting healthy adolescent development;

- care for youth in crisis — strategies for responding through direct assistance to youth in need or crisis;

- advocacy — strategies for challenging systems.

This guide presents research, principles, strategies, and processes for developing intentional pastoral care approaches in youth ministry — relationally and programmatically. Hopefully, you will discover a number of places where you can begin to weave this pastoral care tapestry in your local setting. It is time to make pastoral care a priority in our entire ministry with youth.

ABOUT THE AUTHORS

Michael E. Cavanaugh is a clinical psychologist in private practice and professor of psychology at the University of San Francisco. He is also summer adjunct professor at the Institute of Religious Education and Pastoral Ministry at Boston College. He is the author of *The Effective Minister.*

Joy G. Dryfoos is an independent researcher who has written and lectured extensively on the problems facing youth and families in American today. She is the author of *Adolescents at Risk.*

David A. Hamburg is president of the Carnegie Corporation of New York, one of the country's leading foundations. Educated as a physician, Hamburg has taught at Stanford and Harvard. He is a nationally recognized authority on child development. He is the author of *Today's Children — Creating a Future for a Generation in Crisis.*

Thomas N. Hart teaches theology at Seattle University and is a marriage and family counselor at the Catholic Counseling Center of Seattle. He is the author of several books including *Living Happily Ever After: Toward a Theology of Christian Marriage* and *The Art of Christian Listening.*

Sharon Reed is associate staff member of the Center for Youth Ministry Development and a licensed professional counselor in Columbus, OH. She is a member of the Spirituality Ministry Network in Columbus where she is involved in retreats, workshops and spiritual direction. Sharon also coordinates the supervised ministry component of the Diocesan Lay Ministry Formation Program and is the editor of *Guides to Youth Ministry: Spirituality.*

John Roberto is Director and co-founder of the Center for Youth Ministry Development. John has authored *The Leadership Development Program* (DBM) and has served as editor for a number of DBM publications, including several *Guides to Youth Ministry: Evangelization, Liturgy and Worship, Justice,* and *Early Adolescent Ministry*; and several Catholic Families Series publications: *Growing in Faith: A Catholic*

Families Sourcebook; Media, Faith and Families; Rituals for Sharing Faith; Family Rituals and Celebrations; and *Youth and Families.*

G. Wade Rowatt, Jr. is Professor of Psychology of Religion and Associate Dean of the School of Theology at Southern Baptist Theological Seminary, Louisville. He is the author of *Pastoral Care with Adolescents in Crisis,* a co-author of *The Two Career Marriage* and has written "Caring for the Adolescent in Crisis" (Network Paper 29).

David K. Switzer is Professor of Pastoral Care and Counseling at the Perkins School of Theology, Southern Methodist University, Dallas, Texas. He received a Ph.D. in Theology from Southern California School of Theology. He is the author of *The Dynamics of Grief, The Minister As Crisis Counselor,* and *Pastoral Care Emergencies.* He has been published widely in various journals and contributed to numerous books on the subject of pastoral counseling.

ACKNOWLEDGEMENTS

"Theological Foundations of Pastoral Care" by G. Wade Rowatt, originally appeared as "Adolescents in Crisis" in *Pastoral Care with Adolescents in Crisis* by G. Wade Rowatt (1989). Used by permission of Westminster/John Knox Press.

"The Nature and Scope of Adolescent Problems" by David Hamburg is reprinted from *Today's Children* by David Hamburg (1992). Used by permission of Times Books, a division of Random House, Inc.

"What Does It Mean to Say We Care" and "When and How to Refer" by David Switzer are reprinted from *Pastoral Care Emergencies* by David Switzer (1989). Used by permission of Paulist Press.

"The Psychologically and Pastorally Effective Ministers" by Michael Cavanaugh is reprinted from *The Effective Minister* by Michael Cavanaugh (1986). Used by permission of Harper and Row.

"On Becoming a Helper" by Thomas Hart is reprinted from Chapters 1 and 2 in *The Art of Christian Listening* by Thomas Hart (1980). Used by permission of Paulist Press.

"Common Concepts of Successful Prevention Programs" by Joy G. Dryfoos is excerpted from Chapter 13 of *Adolescents at Risk* by Joy G. Dryfoos (1990). Used by permission of Oxford University Press.

PART I

FOUNDATIONS OF PASTORAL CARE

Overview

In his landmark book, *All Grown Up and No Place To Go,* David Elkind suggested that "the imposition of premature adulthood upon today's teenagers affects them in two different but closely related ways. First, the absence of a protected period of time in which to construct a personal identity impairs the formation of that all important self-definition... The second effect of premature adulthood is inordinate stress." Thus, we have a generation of young people "more vulnerable and less competent to meet the challenges that are inevitable in life" (5). Young people need a place to explore who they are and how they go about nurturing a deeper relationship with their God in the midst of life's struggles. They need the guidance of individuals and a faith community that will advocate for their healthy development in a time whey they are most at-risk.

Guides to Youth Ministry: Pastoral Care attempts to view healthy adolescent development through the lens of pastoral care. In Part I of this book, we pursue the foundational understandings critical to a pastoral care perspective. Part II looks specifically at the pastorally effective minister, and Part III develops practical approaches for integrating pastoral care and youth ministry.

G. Wade Rowatt begins the first part by elaborating the theological foundations of pastoral care. He identifies some of the concerns of today's teens — breakdown of support networks, social problems in their world (AIDS, violence, nuclear war), pressure to succeed, sexuality, and family problems, to name a few. He then examines shepherding as a response to these very real concerns. Scripture is used as a point of reference to bring the adolescent world, revelation, and the faith community together.

In Chapter 2 John Roberto continues this theme as he suggests methods for promoting healthy adolescent development. Using recent research from the Search Institute, Roberto points out the need to develop strategies to develop the internal assets of youth and to strengthen the external support systems in their environment. Even the most resilient young people need the support that pastoral care efforts provide if they are to successfully negotiate adolescence.

David Hamburg then focuses our attention on those young people who may be more at-risk. He reviews the evolution of adolescence and then goes on to survey "the burden of illness, ignorance, and wasted potential." From there Hamburg describes specific problems needing immediate attention: substance abuse, sexuality, depression and suicide, delinquency and violence, divorce. He concludes "To help them learn what they have to learn to survive and flourish and create, we have to understand these circumstances, tasks, and obstacles better than we do now."

Finally in Chapter 4, we return to G. Wade Rowatt for some advice on how to minister to adolescents in crisis. He encourages us to engage ourselves more deeply with adolescents in their world, as participant-observers. He examines the concerns of both early and late adolescence before discussing some basic principles of caring. He divides these into awareness principles and assessment principles. Rowatt concludes with some practical considerations for all those who minister with young people.

CHAPTER 1

THEOLOGICAL FOUNDATIONS OF PASTORAL CARE

G. Wade Rowatt

Caring and counseling, from a religious viewpoint, can best be understood through the image of shepherding. Shepherding is the basic undergirding model for pastoral care and religious counseling (Hiltner). To theoretical foundations drawn from sociology and psychology, shepherding as a theological perspective provides added understanding. This theological dimension primarily distinguishes pastoral care and counseling from other forms of psychotherapy. Trained ministers can be effective psychologists, social workers, and general therapists; when their biblical-theological foundations inform their therapeutic interventions, the care, counseling, or psychotherapy they offer is pastoral.

PASTORAL CARE AS RELATIONSHIP

Pastoral care can be defined as a continuing relationship of support and/or confrontation between a minister and an individual or a group in times of developmental or emergency crisis.[1] Pastoral care is most importantly a relationship. The relationship may be informal, such as casual hallway conversations or across-the-table discussions in a youth lounge, or it may be more formal, "in the office" counseling. In pastoral counseling a specific time, place, and agenda are planned around a therapeutic conversation. In both the formal and informal context the primary key is the relationship. And the relationship is characterized by the shepherding dimension, which will be discussed in more detail in subsequent pages. Pastoral care is with persons, not structural institutions. While social intervention may be a dynamic part of the minister's role, that is outside the scope of care and counseling as defined here. Pastoral care can be with individuals, notably the adolescent in crisis, or with families or groups of adolescents, or with groups of persons important to the adolescent. Pastoral care is not limited to emergencies such as divorce or accident but can also be rendered in developmental crises that emerge as a natural part of the growing process. The birth of a new child may constitute a crisis for the adolescent in that family. Turning sixteen is another developmental crisis.

While professional pastoral care and counseling organizations are twentieth-century phenomena and while research from the behavioral sciences informs modern pastoral care practices, the shepherding stance toward persons in crisis is an ancient biblical concept. Perhaps the shepherding principles are most clearly articulated in Psalm 23 and in Matthew's Gospel (25:40), where Jesus promises that "as you did it to one of the least of these my brethren, you did it to me," as he speaks of the poor, the naked, the sick, the imprisoned, and the hungry. Pastoral care and counseling appear throughout the Scriptures as the shepherding of suffering persons.

Historically, shepherding as a pastoral care perspective developed as a theological dimension in the works of Seward Hiltner, but it has been addressed by many others. An approach that integrates the shepherding perspective of Hiltner with later developments in pastoral care and counseling suggests six interrelated primary dimensions of the shepherding task. These six dimensions — healing, reconciling, sustaining, confronting, guiding, and informing — are woven together in the care and counseling approach to crisis. For the sake of clarity, these dimensions will be analyzed separately; however, in practice one can hardly label a particular ministry response to a crisis as only sustaining or only confronting or only guiding. One of these dimensions may dominate, but the others remain. Caring ministry as a response to crisis reflects some of all six dimensions. The shepherding approach assists persons to face crisis and to experience the richness and fullness of a holistic relationship to themselves, to their environment, and to the future because of the hope they find in God.

DIMENSIONS OF SHEPHERDING

A brief definition of the six dimensions of shepherding is necessary for a discussion of their interrelatedness.

Healing is a process of assisting persons to move toward wholeness, especially in the light of the brokenness brought about by crisis.

Reconciling is a process of assisting persons to move toward restoring wholeness in broken or strained relationships with those who constitute their social environment.

Confronting is a process of moving against the thoughts, feelings, assumptions, or behavioral patterns of persons in response to the crisis.

Sustaining is a process of supporting persons by standing by them and bearing burdens with them while responding to the crisis.

Guiding is a process of assisting persons to make decisions by drawing from within them what was potentially available in their own decision-making.

Informing is a process of clarifying alternatives for persons by providing specific new information and data.

Healing and Reconciling

The foundational question in a shepherding response to crisis involves a polarity between healing and reconciling. What is the goal? The crisis caregiver or counselor holds healing and reconciliation in dynamic tension and responds by suggesting the possibilities of both. While healing is the ultimate goal for the individual in crisis, reconciling is the primary objective for the individual's relationships to others in the crisis. Both find significance as shepherding ministry from the biblical perspective.

The four Gospels record 26 cases, excluding the parallels, of individuals who were healed by Jesus. The language of salvation itself blends with the language of healing throughout the New Testament. Jesus frequently intertwined the dimensions of physical healing and personal wholeness or salvation in his ministry, for instance, as he healed the man sick of palsy who was lowered through the roof in the midst of the crowd (Mark 2:1-2). Jesus performed the healing miracle there as a prerequisite for the faith necessary for wholeness and salvation. Also in the epistles, Paul's work in healing supports the view of the early Christians that physical and spiritual wholeness are interwoven.

Ministers concerned with healing and reconciliation with adolescents in crisis are cautioned to avoid two common errors. On the one hand, they might inappropriately push the question of the adolescent's relationship to God in a way that angers the adolescent enough to break the counseling relationship and terminate further caregiving. However, on the other hand, they need to avoid the assumption that no examination of faith is appropriate. A crisis will raise questions of one's faith stance (particularly in reflecting). Ultimate questions for reflection come after the crisis has passed its critical point and will focus around one's relationships, around one's view of self, and around the future. These each have a theological dimension. Relationship to the self begins with a belief in the goodness (or the evil) of creation and continues with understanding the meaning of redemption and incarnation. The relationship to self is ultimately asked: "Am I a person of worth, created in the image of God, loved by God, and therefore of value?" Questions about relationships are basically faith queries. "Can one's environment be trusted? Are the powers of light able to sustain the battle against the powers of darkness?" The response of persons of faith is that "the light shines in the darkness, and the darkness has not overcome it" (John 1:5). Facing one's environment is ultimately a question of faith. Facing the future is fundamentally a theological question of hope. The foundation of hope from a religious perspective is in the working of a Being greater than all personhood, but it is not devoid of the responsibility of persons and the goodness of persons. While ministers are cautioned against prematurely and inappropriately pushing religious questions into a crisis situation, they must also be cautioned not to ignore the impact of faith questions on the response to the crisis.

Healing of the person is a primary goal, but healing cannot be understood apart from reconciliation with one's environment. No person can be whole and remain isolated from meaningful relatedness. Crises can result from broken relationships, but more frequently they produce broken relationship.

Reconciliation, a major theme of Christian Scripture, is a process of restoring broken or strained relationships between persons, individuals, and God. Reconciliation is bridge-building over the troubled waters of crisis. Reconciliation is the caring minister's response to disunity and brokenness. The incarnation has at its heart reconciling persons to God. Paul appeals for reconciliations many times but most notably in the dispute over the differentness of spiritual gifts (1 Cor. 12:21-26). Shepherding as a ministry of reconciliation attempts to assist adolescents to see their place in the family, with their peers, and in society at large and to equip them to live in growing, mutually enhancing relationships.

Reconciliation, built upon several theological themes, involves awareness of the brokenness, confession of one's own participation in the brokenness, however large or small that might seem, and the giving and receiving of forgiveness. Sometimes a ritual of acceptance such as the verbal pronouncement of a blessing on the adolescent serves as a powerful symbol of reconciliation in times of crisis. However, most often a hug, a handshake, a gift, or a shared moment of laughter becomes the unlabeled ritual of reconciliation.

Confronting and Sustaining

Healing the self and reconciling with the environment remain in tension as the shepherd responds to a crisis. Two relationship stances can be taken toward both healing and reconciliation. They are confronting and sustaining. These two stances must also be held in dynamic tension.

Like healing and reconciling, confronting and sustaining are biblical models for a shepherding ministry. Confronting is the application of the law, while sustaining is more an expression of grace. Confronting occurs throughout the Scriptures and can mean moving against the environment as well as against a person's assumptions, thoughts, feelings, or behavioral patterns. The prophets spoke boldly, not only to individuals, as in the confrontation of King David for his involvement with Bathsheba, but also to environments, as the prophets Jeremiah and Amos spoke to the culture of their time.

Furthermore, in Matthew's Gospel, Jesus provides a model for confronting. In Matthew 18:15-22, the disciples are instructed to confront a "brother" if they feel wronged by him. Jesus' model of individual, personal confrontation sets the goal of dealing with one's self confessionally and being restored to wholeness with one's environment. If the confrontation cannot be handled individually in dealing with the self, others are involved until the confrontation is resolved or the individual is excluded from the group. With adolescents and broken family relationships, there is a time when out-of-home placements and changing environments is the ultimate theological response.

Jesus confronted not only individuals but also the culture of his time, seeking reconciliation between individuals and their environment. You can see as Jesus speaks to oppressed and persecuted persons (such as the woman taken in adultery) that he seeks reconciliation in the environment. Paul, reflecting upon this ministry, writes in Galatians 3:28 that in Christ there is no male or female, no Jew or Greek, no bond or free. Confrontation has its ultimate goal — total reconciliation and healing.

Ministers must be careful to note that the authority of confrontation does not come from one's own personality and perceived superior ability but from one's role as a representative of the congregation, the society, and the word of God. The authority and privilege of confrontation are expressed as the representative of something larger than one's self. We must take care not to risk rejecting individuals through unrealistic private confrontations. Ultimately, the confrontation should be such that persons feel they have encountered a truth larger than themselves and the individual with whom they speak. The truth of confrontation produces hope when shared in the context of love.

Sustaining exists in dynamic tension with confrontation as the fourth shepherding dimension. Sustaining, like confrontation, is an approach of bringing wholeness to a self and reconciliation to the environment. Sustaining consists of supporting persons by standing by them in their quest for healing and reconciliation. Understanding, feeling with, and accepting an individual moves them toward wholeness and is at the heart of the sustaining process.

The sustaining aspect of shepherding is also seen throughout the Old and New Testaments. God is with the bewildered and lost slaves in Egypt and sustains them in their pilgrimage through the wilderness as they move toward their future in the promised land. Galatians 6:2 admonishes Christians to "bear one another's burdens." Sustaining, a continuing process of seeking to preserve hope, encourages self-acceptance. In the face of a crisis, adolescents sometimes overgeneralize and magnify problems out of proportion. Sustaining teens as individuals maintains a degree of self-respect and hope.

In a time of crisis, sustaining the environment may also be needed. The adolescent's parents, siblings, extended family, peers, and perhaps teachers and others all need a word of encouragement from the caregiver. The caregiver can be an advocate for the adolescent, thus sustaining efforts toward reconciliation in the present or at some point in the future.

Confronting and sustaining are maintained in tension without either excluding the other from the context of caregiving. Wayne Oates uses the analogy of hand surgery in discussing his approach to shepherding. Early hand surgeons would literally hold the hand of the patient in one hand while performing the surgery with their other hand. The underneath hand symbolizing the sustaining, while the hand with the surgical instrument represents the confrontation. Both are necessary.

In a team approach to adolescent ministry, it is not unusual for some members to take a confrontive, hard-line, maintain-the-rules, administrative approach to a given adolescent in crisis, while other members of the team take a supportive, understanding, "I'm-your-friend" approach. These representations of law and grace are easier to make when a team is responding to the crisis, but sometimes both must be made by one person. A single caregiver can maintain the tension between confronting and sustaining as the process of responding to the crisis unfolds.

Guiding and Informing

A third set of shepherding polarities, guiding and informing, are similarly to be held in tension. Both guiding and informing are perspectives for confronting and sustaining, which are in turn perspectives for healing and reconciling. An attempt to provide new information produces the confrontation. At other times, guiding the person's thoughts, and reflections leads to self-confrontation. Likewise, in sustaining individuals and environments, informing will be the approach at times. In other situations, guiding individuals to examine their own thoughts and reflections will lead to sustaining.

Like confronting, sustaining, reconciling, and healing, guiding has its foundation in Christian Scripture. Guiding is seen throughout the Old Testament, where both the prophets and the priests proclaim and teach the word of God in hope of a response from their listeners. Furthermore, as Jesus talks with the accusers about to stone the woman taken in adultery, he draws out to them the criteria for making their decision. In John 8:7 he demands, "Let him who is without sin among you be the first to throw a stone." As the hearers reflect on the implications of his statement, they turn one at a time to leave. They have been guided in the process of making their own decision, never directly informed of the decision Jesus would have made.

Guiding (this process of helping persons discover within themselves the resources for making decisions) involves reflection upon thoughts, feelings, attitudes, and behaviors. Adolescents in particular may need assistance in differentiating between their thoughts, feelings, and attitudes. *Feeling Good* by David Burns provides excellent information in the process of examining and differentiating thoughts, feelings, and attitudes. [2] Guiding is an integral part of shepherding ministry when choices are offered by the person in crisis and examined in light of their understanding of potential outcomes. In direct contrast to guiding, informing brings information from outside the individual to bear upon confrontation and sustaining.

Informing, a process of clarifying alternatives by providing specific new information, also has a broad foundation in Christian Scripture. In Isaiah 40:28-31 the prophet questions his listeners: "Have you not known? Have you not heard? The Lord is the everlasting God. He does not faint or grow weary.... Even youths shall faint and be weary....; but they who wait for the Lord shall renew their strength, they shall mount up with wings like eagles, they shall run and not be weary, they shall walk and not faint." This information is provided as a form of sustaining individuals and their environment in a time of crisis.

In the New Testament we see an example of informing as a means of sustaining individuals and confronting their time of grief when Paul, writing to the church at Thessalonica (1 Thess. 4:16), addresses their concern for Christians who have died before Christ's return. Their grief over the loss of their fellow Christians is both confronted and sustained by Paul as he writes, "The dead in Christ will rise first." The shepherding response of informing involves input of new data.

Informing has long been a part of Christian ministry, but it has not regularly been incorporated in shepherding. The teaching and preaching ministries of the church have highlighted the imparting of new information. However, shepherding, caregiving, and counseling can also be avenues of providing new information. Perhaps in the way questions are asked, information voids can be revealed and appropriate responses made. For example, a young man in a substance-abuse crisis can be asked about the substance's effects and then information provided if he does not have accurate data. Informing may take the part of educating adolescents as to the consequences of their behavior or pointing them toward information from other resources that can be applied in a particular crisis.

In summary, shepherding ministry has as its primary goal bringing wholeness to individuals and reconciliation to their environment in a context of hope. Frequently, confronting and sustaining are relationship stances between the counselor, the individual, and the environment. Informing and guiding are perspectives for confronting and sustaining and likewise are to be held in dynamic tension.

End Notes

[1]Oates, Wayne E. *New Dimensions in Pastoral Care.* Philadelphia, PA: Fortress Press, 1970.

[2]Burns, David D. *Feeling Good: The New Mood Therapy.* New York, NY: Signet Books, 1981.

Works Cited

Clebsch, William A. and Charles R. Jaekle. *Pastoral Care in Historical Perspective.* Englewood Cliffs, NJ: Prentice-Hall, 1964.

Hiltner, Seward. *Preface to Pastoral Theology.* Nashville, TN: Convention Press, 1977.

Oates, Wayne. *Pastoral Counseling.* Philadelphia, PA: Westminster Press, 1974.

CHAPTER 2

PROMOTING HEALTHY ADOLESCENT DEVELOPMENT

John Roberto

Promoting the healthy development of youth presents a tremendous challenge for all youth-serving institutions in our society today. From local community, religious, and educational institutions to the government and national organizations, the concern for positive youth development is growing. We are all alarmed by the staggering number of our young people whose journey from childhood to adult maturity is at-risk from factors such as poverty, poor education, or anti-social behaviors such as drugs or alcohol abuse, and unsafe sexual activity.

What role can churches play in promoting healthy adolescent development? This is the question that guides this essay. We start our analysis with the reality of adolescent development today. We then explore a model of healthy adolescent development, and conclude with strategies and suggestions for promoting positive youth development.

THE REALITY AND HOPE

The National Commission on Children in their report, *Beyond Rhetoric*, reported that the majority of young people emerge from adolescence healthy, hopeful, and able to meet the challenges to adult life. Half of America's 10- to 17-year-olds are doing well and are at very low risk of experiencing problems related to their social behavior. They are progressing in school, they are not sexually active, they do not commit delinquent acts, and they do not use drugs or alcohol.

Approximately one-quarter of young people are at moderate risk of experiencing problems: they are doing less well in school and may be behind a grade or more; if they are sexually active they are likely to use contraception; they experiment with alcohol or drugs occasionally; and some commit minor delinquent offenses. Most of these young people will become responsible adults and will not suffer any lasting harm, although they will experience some problems and adjustments along the way.

One-quarter of American adolescents engage in high-risk behaviors that endanger their own health and well-being and that of others as well. These seven million young people have multiple problems that can severely limit their futures: most have fallen far behind in school, and some have already dropped out; they engage in unprotected sexual activity, and some have experienced pregnancies or contracted sexually transmitted diseases; some have been arrested or have committed serious offenses; and typically they are frequent and heavy users of drugs and alcohol.

Complicating this portrait is the reality that at every age, among all races and income groups, and in communities nationwide, many youth are in jeopardy from forces in their communities. Many young people grow up in families whose lives are in turmoil. Their parents are too stressed and too drained to provide the nurture, structure, and security that protect children and prepare them for adulthood. Some of these young people are unloved and neglected. Others are unsafe at home and in their neighborhoods. Many are poor and some are homeless and hungry. Often they lack the rudiments of basic health care and a quality education. Almost always, they lack hope and dreams, a vision of what their lives can become, and the support and guidance to make it a reality. [1]

The reality of growing up in America today poses a dilemma for churches and those who minister with youth. Many will see this portrait and focus on what is wrong with young people today. This is an attitude that is all too prevalent in our society, and in many churches. Peter Scales summarizes such a view when he writes,

When we do pay attention to young adolescents, the frame of reference often used is a problem, such as adolescent pregnancy, substance abuse, or school dropout, rather than the whole adolescent. We view young people in a splintered and fragmented way, as a collection of discrete problems, to be responded to by an equally fragmented system of education, health, and social services. While some insist that genuine prevention of the problems of young adolescents requires a looking at young people holistically and arranging support systems comprehensively, others take refuge in inertia, which remains a powerful force (Scales 6-7.)

If we are to promote successfully the healthy growth and development of all adolescents, we must focus not on what is wrong with adolescents, but rather on what is right. We need to build on their strengths.

While we all too often see the negative picture of adolescents in our society, we do not as readily see a picture of positive possibilities, of the majority of adolescents who are not falling victim to risky behaviors. In this picture, 80% of young people are happy with their family lives, 70% of 15 year-olds have not had sexual intercourse, 80% of young people under 17 do not have a drinking problem, and 80% are not regular smokers, among other facts. The picture is there, but we only perceive it faintly, like the good news and decent acts of humanity that occur in our lives but that we tend to assume are rare (Scales 7).

We must view adolescents through the lens of *positive possibilities.* I prefer an approach which builds on the strengths of adolescents, their families and communities, while admitting that struggles and problems are clearly a part of the adolescent experience. Churches that adopt this stance see themselves in the "business" of promoting healthy adolescent development through everything they do. They take an active stance and seek ways to partner with families and community agencies in a common effort. Churches have not always thought of themselves as a community organization that is in the "business" of promoting healthy adolescent development, but that *is* what they do. The challenge is for churches to take more seriously their role in positive youth development. Churches have resources, experience, commitments, and values that can greatly contribute to healthy adolescent development. They provide an intergenerational community in which healthy relationships and a sense of belonging can be nurtured. Most importantly, churches have a faith tradition that provides a solid foundation upon which to build a healthy identity and lifestyle.

This essay will focus on positive youth development. *Positive youth development is best described as the process through which adolescents actively seek, and are assisted, to meet their basic needs and build their individual assets or competencies.* This is one of the three elements of pastoral care. It is important to remember that the pastoral care of adolescents includes two other interdependent elements: *caring for youth in crisis* — responding through direct assistance to youth at risk or in need, and *advocacy* — challenging social systems (government, education) to promote to more effectively address youth issues and promote positive youth development.

A MODEL OF HEALTHY ADOLESCENT DEVELOPMENT

In *The Troubled Journey: A Profile of American Youth,* Peter Benson of the Search Institute suggests a very helpful way to view adolescent development. [2] *The Troubled Journey* reveals two important groups of factors that promote healthy development and reduce the likelihood of adolescents' participation in behavior that puts them at risk. One group identifies *assets external to the adolescent,* but present in family and community. Another group identifies *strengths to be found within the adolescent.* Benson writes,

> When children are growing up, the kind of help they most need is usually supplied by a combination of the family and the surrounding community. The family provides rules, discipline, encouragement, and caring. The community makes available such things as educational experiences, community rules and expectations, friends, recreational experiences, and spiritual nurture. These are the external assets.
>
> These external assets, taken together, form a kind of temporary scaffold around a child in order to support and encourage while the growing child is developing an internal system of supports that will see him or her safely into adulthood. Their function is much like that of the scaffolds built around buildings during erection or repair to provide a temporary stability until the building is ready to stand on its own. They are there to do what needs to be done while young people are developing their own internal supports — until they develop *backbone* (April 1991 *Source* 1).

In a perfect world young people's internal strengths would develop gradually throughout adolescence, while external supports were being removed at the same gradual rate. The research shows, however, that while some internal strengths increase during the teen years, too often the external assets are being removed before adequate internal strength development occurs.

The images of *scaffold* and *backbone* go a long way toward capturing the dynamics of growth during adolescence. Promoting healthy growth involves providing a supportive community for youth — external support and care, *and* assisting young people to develop their identity, values, and faith life — internal assets or strengths. Research points to a number of important interventions we can make in our work with youth to promote healthy development. I have listed a number of these interventions that can make a *big* difference in the lives of youth in the last section of this essay.

The Search Institute study is not alone in its conclusions. Major research studies all point to the necessity of developing the coping skills, social supports, and self-esteem of adolescents. What they also point to, and what contemporary policy recommendations are coming to reflect, is that young people live in a complex context of families, schools, and communities. The efforts that have the greatest chance of promoting well-being among young people are those that recognize this reality and consciously try to develop partnerships among schools, families, churches, and community organizations.

In light of this I would like to propose a model for viewing adolescent development, which builds upon the interplay of external support and structure — supplied by family, school, church, and responsive community organizations — and the development of an internal system of assets, competencies, and skills that will see the adolescent safely into adulthood. I am aware of the dangers and criticisms inherent in suggesting an optimal model of development. Many will think that proposing such a model is naive or idealistic, given the reality of the problems facing youth as they grow into adulthood. (In Chapter 3 of this book David Hamburg describes many of the obstacles that hinder healthy development.) Unless we know what factors work together to promote optimal growth we will have great difficulty developing approaches and strategies that promote positive youth development.

At the center of the model is our understanding of the growth characteristics of adolescents which comes to us from psycho-social, moral, and faith development research. These *life changes* and *developmental needs* give us insights into the internal dynamics of growth during adolescence. They permeate the adolescent experience, providing clues into the what and how of positive development. They give us the basis of responding effectively to the needs and interests of adolescents, creating developmentally appropriate strategies and programs. While this research is extremely helpful in describing the journey and providing direction for ministry, it must be remembered that the adolescent is far more complex and mysterious than these descriptions of life tasks and needs.

Drawn from our understanding of the developmental needs of adolescents are specific *internal assets.* These include positive commitments, values, attitudes, and social competencies necessary for healthy growth into adulthood. The development of these internal assets are dependent to a large degree on the *external supports* of family, church, school, and community organizations. They provide networks of care, support, and structure for the young person as he or she develops internal strengths throughout adolescence.

A Model of Healthy Adolescent Development

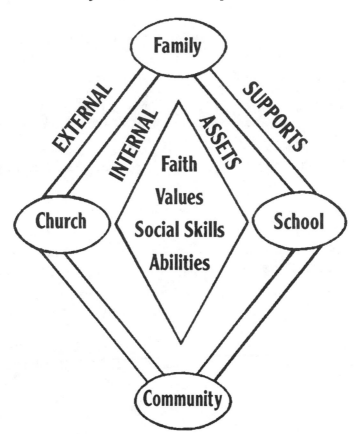

We turn our attention first to the developmental tasks and needs of young and older adolescents. Using the research from the Search Institute's *Troubled Journey* study, we will identify the internal assets and external supports necessary for healthy growth.

Developmental Tasks and Needs of Adolescents

Early Adolescent Growth

With the exception of infancy, no time in life compresses more physical, intellectual, social, emotional, moral and faith development into so brief a span. Briefly summarized, the key changes of early adolescence (10-14/15 year olds) involve:

- experiencing rapid physical growth including the development of secondary sex characteristics and the capacity to reproduce;

- moving from concrete thinking (what is) to abstract thinking (what might be true if...);

- constructing a consistent self-image and discovering who they are as unique persons;

- engaging in more complex decision-making;

- redefining their relationship with family and moving toward limited autonomy while still looking to family for affection and guidance in setting values;

- identifying more strongly with the peer group for belonging and deepening friendships;

- establishing a set of religious beliefs, attitudes and values grounded in family *and* in a caring faith community.

Table 1 in the *Appendix* presents a more extended overview of the developmental changes that take place during early adolescence. [3]

The developmental needs of young adolescents arise out of these changes. They provide a very useful framework for understanding the positive possibilities of early adolescence, thereby providing a solid basis upon which to build ministry strategies and programming. The following chart describes the eight developmental needs of young adolescents.

THE DEVELOPMENTAL NEEDS OF YOUNG ADOLESCENTS

Opportunities for Young Adolescents:

Self-Definition

- to better understand, define, and accept who they are as individuals

- to explore their widening social world and to reflect upon the meaning of new experiences, so that they can consider themselves participants in society

- to achieve a positive orientation toward the mainstream American culture and their own minority culture; to affirm their ethnicity through observation of ceremonies, retention of native language, and reinforcement of specific attitudes, beliefs, and practices

Competence and Achievement

- to find out what they are good at doing and to know what they do is valued by others whom they respect

- to encourage the practice of new skills, public performance and recognition, and reflection on personal and group accomplishments

Positive Social Interaction with Adults and Peers

- to develop interpersonal skills

- to learn how to develop a relationship with their parents that is reflective of their growing autonomy and utilizes new patterns of communicating

- to form positive peer relationships and support, especially through structured programs

- to form caring relationships with adults who like and respect them, who share their own experiences, views, values, and feelings, and who serve as role models and advisors

Meaningful Participation in Families, Schools, Churches and Community Organizations

- to participate in making decisions about activities that shape their lives *and* as active leaders or participants who can make a viable contribution to the success of those activities

- to participate as valued members of the faith community and as leaders in church ministries and programs

- to make available situations in which they can use their skills to solve real life problems and affect the world around them, such as community service programs

Physical Activity

- to utilize their energy and growing bodies through activities that require physical movement or expression

Creative Expression

- to express to the external world who they are on the inside (feelings, interests, abilities, thoughts) through a variety of activities, e.g. music, writing, sports, art, drama, cooking

- to afford activities that enable them to experience and test out new and different forms of self-expression

Personal Religious Experience

- to explore "the big questions" in life, questions whose answers can only be comprehended within the context of faith and religion

- to promote occasions for a deeper and more personal relationship with God

Structure and Clear Limits

- to provide structure and guidance for young adolescents in making decisions about their behavior that involve them in the process of decision-making

- to put in place structure that helps them stay focused on a task, persevere in their various efforts and succeed, which leads to an increase in self-esteem

- to define clearly structure and limits that help them feel safe in their activities, which can empower them to live with joy and confidence

Older Adolescent Growth

Older adolescent growth must be seen as an ongoing process beginning around the first years of high school and culminating in the years after graduation. Briefly summarized, the key changes of older adolescents, aged 15-18/19, involve:

• reaching adult growth and sexual maturity;

• developing the ability to engage in reflective thinking about what they know, value, and believe ("what do I think?" and "why do I think that?");

• beginning the process of establishing a personal identity, a meaningful self-concept, which includes an acceptance of one's sexuality, vocational goals, and philosophy of life;

• shifting from inherited authority (especially the family) to self-chosen authority (eventually oneself), often by establishing an identity that is powerfully shaped by significant others (peers and adults);

• reevaluating the moral values received from family, church, and significant others (adults, peers) and searching for a moral code which preserves their personal integrity and provides the basis for developing an internalized moral value system that can guide their behavior;

• moving toward greater personal intimacy and adult sexuality;

• developing the capability for more mutual, trusting, deep, and enduring personal friendships with members of the same sex and opposite sex;

• expanding their perspective to encompass the motives, feelings, and thought patterns of individuals and groups of peoples outside their personal experience;

• exploring and questioning the faith handed down by family and church as they search for a style of faith and belief which is more personal to them.

Table 2 in the *Appendix* presents a more extended overview of the developmental changes that take place during older adolescence. [4]

The developmental needs of older adolescents arise out of these changes. They serve as a very useful framework for understanding the positive possibilities of older adolescence, thereby providing a solid basis upon which to build ministry strategies and programming. The following chart describes several of the developmental needs of older adolescents.

DEVELOPMENTAL NEEDS OF OLDER ADOLESCENTS

Opportunities for Older Adolescents:

Exploration and Experimentation

- to experiment with a wide array of behaviors, roles, attitudes, relationships, ideas, and activities as they develop their own identity and faith identity

- to explore who they are and who they can become by reflecting on self in relation to others

- to achieve a positive orientation toward the dominant American culture and their own minority culture; to affirm their ethnicity through observation of ceremonies, retention of native language, and reinforcement of specific attitudes, beliefs, and practices

Adult Sexuality

- to understand sexual growth and integrate sexuality into their personality in a holistic way

- to develop healthy values and attitudes regarding their own sexuality

Interpersonal Relationships

- to form positive relationships and experiences with peers in a comfortable and secure environment and to develop friendship-making and friendship-maintaining skills

- to learn how to develop a relationship with parents that is reflective of their growing autonomy and utilizes new patterns of communicating

Meaningful Roles in the Community and Society

- to participate with other older adolescents as full members and leaders in the community, society and church

- to explore, discuss, and act on local and global justice issues; to develop an active responsibility for what happens in their community and world, and to be involved in meaningful community service

• to be involved in the decision-making, planning, and implementation of programs that serve them

Preparing for the Future

• to acquire the competencies necessary for adult roles, such as goal setting, problem solving, time management, and decision making

• to explore life options and plan their futures (career, education) and to help them acquire the skills, knowledge and experience for their chosen fields; to link more closely the worlds of school and work

Personal Value System and Decision-Making Skills

• to discuss conflicting values and formulate their own value system

• to gain knowledge and experience in making decisions and to apply Christian moral values in making moral judgments

Personal Faith

• to explore and question the faith they have been given by family and the faith community and develop their own faith identity

• to explore what it means to be and live as a person of faith today

• to develop a more personal relationship with Jesus Christ

Adult Mentors

• to develop relationships with adult Christians who affirm their journey and struggles, explore sensitive issues with them, listen to their stories and questions, share their own faith journey, and ask questions that encourage critical thinking and reflection

DEVELOPING THE STRENGTHS OF ADOLESCENTS

We now turn our attention to the internal assets or strengths that we want to promote in the lives of young people. As already cited, *The Troubled Journey: A Profile of American Youth* identifies 14 essential elements of the internal supports that make positive growth possible for teenagers. Thirteen of the fourteen are positive, a listing of values, attitudes, and skills that caring adults hope young people develop during their adolescent years. They are divided into three categories: commitment to education, positive values, and social competence. Only one (values sexual restraint) implies a "just say no" message. [5]

External Assets

Educational Commitment

The first essential component of internal support is enthusiasm for the educational process, now and well into the future. Four elements were identified in the study:

1. *School Performance*: working at or above average performance
2. *Achievement Motivation*: caring about their school performance and wanting to do well
3. *Homework*: spending six or more hours each week on homework
4. *Educational Aspiration*: hoping to go on after high school to college or technical school

Positive Values

The second essential component of internal support is positive values — values that center on caring about others as well as oneself. Four elements were identified in the study:

5. *Values Sexual Restraint*: postponing sexual activity as a personal goal, "just say no"
6. *Values Helping People*: being of help to others
7. *Is Concerned About World Hunger and Poverty*: expressing a desire to better the circumstances of those who are hungry and in poverty
8. *Cares About Other People's Feelings*: attending to the well-being of others

Social Competence

The third essential component of internal support is social competence and social skills — success in interacting with others, in learning how to work in groups, in "holding your own" against opposition, and in anticipating what is coming. Six elements were identified in the study:

9. *Self Esteem:* having a reasonable sense of one's own value
10. *Assertiveness Skills*: standing up for what one believes — explaining your understandings and needs clearly and firmly, without being angry or abrasive in doing so
11. *Decision-making Skills*: dealing with increasingly complex decisions
12. *Friend-making Skills*: mastering the skills for making and keeping friends
13. *Planning Skills*: being able to map out one's future over the next days, months or years and being able to delay what seems most attractive right now in order to complete the less-desirable but necessary task
14. *Positive View of Personal Future*: feeling positive about the future and their own future

If we focus on positive values and social competence and the elements associated with each of these components, it should be clear that churches can play a very important role in developing these assets through programs and activities. It should also be evident that the Christian faith is a tremendous resource in promoting healthy development. The Christian faith provides a value base from which young people can develop the positive values outlined above, such as valuing sexual restraint, helping or prosocial behaviors, caring about others. The Christian value system also provides a basis for developing social competence, especially in responsible decision-making and developing a positive view of the future. Youth who decide not to engage in negative behaviors often do so because of their value system.

There are two challenges that churches face in promoting internal assets. First, it involves designing or redesigning existing programming to promote these 14 assets intentionally. Secondly, it requires finding people and other resources that address from a values context the "real life" issues youth face, many of which are at-risk issues. It is critical that the Christian faith gives new meaning to the "real life" issues youth face. Indeed, young people's long-term involvement in and loyalty toward faith institutions may be dependent on whether their congregations address these issues. If not, young people may see faith institutions, finally, as irrelevant — a pattern and a memory that is no longer significant.

DEVELOPING COMMUNITY SUPPORTS

To this point we have focused primarily on the growing adolescent and the assets necessary for growth into adulthood. It is time to focus our attention on the broader community and its role in providing the external supports for the growth process. The 14 internal characteristics combine with 16 external assets to make up a network of interior and exterior strengths that has remarkable power to *shield* adolescents against at-risk behaviors and *promote* positive teenage development. They equip adolescents to make wise choices.

One of the major contributions of the *The Troubled Journey: A Profile of American Youth* is that it identifies those elements in the family and in the community that appear, in effect, to protect teenagers against the kinds of trouble most feared by parents, teachers, and others who work with adolescents. The more assets a teenager reports being present in his or her life, the fewer the at-risk behaviors that teenager displays.

These 16 external assets provide the kinds of interest, care, and structure that are essential if an adolescent is to progress through the teenage years relatively untroubled. They supply a necessary network of support while adolescents develop internal supports firm enough to carry them successfully into adult life. Eight of these external assets lie mostly within the control of individual families. The remaining eight are community-based, requiring the cooperation or initiative of persons or groups outside the family. Thus it is evident that neither the community nor the family can assume the entire responsibility for the support of adolescents. They must work together. [6]

External Assets

Support

The first essential component of external assets is support, creating an atmosphere of appreciation and encouragement that provides young people with experiences of being loved, successful, and worthwhile. Thus equipped, one can survive the inevitable temporary failures and defeats of daily life. Of the seven external assets included under external assets: support, the first four assets are almost entirely family-generated and the remaining three depend largely on institutions outside the family.

1. *Family Support*: providing high levels of love and support

2. *Parent(s) as Social Resource*: viewing parents as people one can go to for advice, comfort, and encouragement

3. *Parent Communication*: having frequent, in-depth conversation with parents

4. *Parent Involvement in Schooling*: continuing to show interest in the nature of their children's school work and success in school

5. *Other Adult Communication*: having frequent, in-depth conversations with adults other than parents

6. *Other Adult Resources*: knowing non-parent adults to go to for advice and support

7. *Positive School Climate*: caring, encouraging school environment

Control

The second essential component of external assets is controls on behavior — learning how to exercise some self-discipline, to develop will power to complete projects, to allocate time to life's demands according to carefully-thought-through priorities rather than momentary impulse. These are essential capacities that most adults absorbed by having certain controls imposed throughout adolescence. While the first four elements of this category are largely parent-controlled, the final one is related to circumstances largely beyond family control.

8. *Parental Standards*: making expectations of behavior and the penalties for inappropriate behavior known to adolescents

9. *Parental Discipline*: disciplining adolescents for violating family rules

10. *Parental Monitoring*: knowing where the adolescent is going when he or she leaves the house, with whom, and for approximately how long

11. *Time at Home*: insuring that the adolescent goes out for fun and recreation no more than three nights a week

12. *Positive Peer Influence*: developing friends who approve of and model responsible behavior

Structured Use of Time

The third essential component of external assets is the development of a disciplined structure — working at a task to meet given deadlines, not at one's own convenience or whim. Four elements fit into this category of external assets. All of them, though partly dependent on family decision, largely depend on activities provided and supervised for youth by adult members of the community.

13. *Involved in Music*: spending one hour or more per week in music training or practice

14. *Involved in School Extra-curricular Activities*: spending one hour or more each week participating in school-related sports, clubs, or organizations

15. *Involved in Community Organizations or Activities*: spending an hour or more each week participating in organizations or clubs outside of school

16. *Involved in Church or Synagogue Activities*: spending an hour or more per week attending worship services or participating in church activities

In addition to the 16 external assets identified in *The Troubled Journey* study, we can focus on the important role that the faith of the family and the congregation provides to this external system of support and care. A strong family faith life nurtures greater faith maturity in adolescents. Parents can influence the faith maturity of adolescents in three significant ways: 1) through modeling and personal example — when parents talk about their actions and when what they say is consistent with what they do; 2) through agreement — when parents agree on the importance of religion to them and the messages they convey are consistent, and 3) through discussion — when parents talk at home about religious activity and motivation(Williams).

The type of congregational life that young people experience is extremely important for promoting healthy development. In fact, *The Troubled Journey* study reports that youth who attended religious services at least once or twice a month were nearly half as likely to engage in any of the at-risk behaviors than those who rarely or never attended religious services. Churches can promote greater maturity of faith and stronger congregational and denominational loyalty in youth in several significant ways: 1) through effective Christian education; 2) through a congregational climate that is a warm and friendly community and that encourages questions, challenges thinking, and expects learning; 3) through quality worship; 4) through service to those in need; 5) through experiencing the care and concern of other members; 6) through promoting active participation of all members in parish life and encouraging each member to take responsibility for some part of the parish's life, and 7) through effective leadership which demonstrates concern and affirmation(Benson and Eklin).

The model of adolescent development proposed in this essay is intended to provide a holistic view of healthy adolescent development. It points us toward a ministry with youth which provides developmentally appropriate programs and activities, cultivates the internal assets of youth, strengthens family life, incorporates young people into church life, and partners with schools, churches, and community organizations in a common efforts on behalf of youth. Using this holistic model, we now turn to practical strategies for promoting positive youth development.

BECOMING A RESPONSIVE COMMUNITY

Organizational Strategies for Positive Youth Development

In a youth-centered America, every community would have a network of affordable, accessible, safe, and challenging opportunities that appeal to the diverse interests of adolescents. Youth development services would provide meaningful opportunities for young people to pursue individual interests as well as to contribute to their communities. They would grant youth appropriate degrees of autonomy. They would be organized through responsive program, organizational, and community structures. They would be rooted in a solid foundation of research- and practice-based knowledge of the needs of children and adolescents and supported by a dependable and diverse financial base. Finally, they would be grounded on suggestions from youth themselves (*A Matter of Time* 77).

This is the vision of community support that we want to strengthen and create. *Community support means building a range of formal and informal structures that surround, encourage, and protect young people and their families.* Both accepted theory and empirical evidence strongly support the idea that community-based programs are essential to the healthy development of adolescents (*A Matter of Time*).

The challenge for churches is simple but not easy. Churches must begin to think in terms of youth development and view themselves in the broader context of community supports consisting of families, schools, organizations, and other faith institutions. The summary of developmental needs of young and older adolescents and the internal assets and external supports point to the necessary ingredients of positive development. The strategies outlined below build on the research and suggest practical approaches that seek to prevent deficits and to promote assets. The list is not exhaustive; it is meant to stimulate your own creativity. Remember that there are a large number of resources to help you in your work. A bibliography in the last chapter of this book correlates resource with strategies. Be sure to inventory the resources in your community: people, programs, organizations, print and audio-visual materials.

Strategy 1: Promote Positive Values

In order to provide young people with a solid values basis for their lives, we need to promote positive, life-giving values that center on caring about others as well as oneself, such as serving others, caring about other people's feelings and attending to their well-being, concern for betterment of life for all people, and valuing sexual restraint. Stated another way, we need to promote Gospel values in all programs and relationships. Gospel values, such as compassion, honesty, integrity, human dignity, equality, and service to others all contribute to a solid foundation upon which to build one's life. A first step in implementing this strategy is evaluate *all* youth ministry programming to discover the values that are being communicated explicitly and implicitly and to strengthen the positive values base of every program and activity.

Strategy 2: Develop Life Skills

One of the most significant ways to promote positive youth development is by creating intentional programs and activities which develop the life skills of adolescents. Adolescents need to learn how to make decisions, how to communicate with others, how to make friends, how to stand up for what they believe, how to resolve conflicts nonviolently, how to negotiate, how to solve problems, how to think critically, how to plan, how to get things done, and how to interpret media and its many images and messages. They need to learn responsibility and self-control. They also need opportunities to deal directly with important adolescent struggles and to discuss these issues and the feelings they generate. A life skills curriculum must be skills-based and highly experiential. A youth ministry can become a laboratory where youth practice the how-to's of life as well as the how-to's of the Christian faith.

Every church should sponsor life skills training as a integral part of their youth ministry or religious education programming. You can sponsor separate courses or workshops, or integrate life skills training in other program formats. There are several life skills programs already created that you can use. Investigate what churches, schools and other youth organizations in community are already doing. You might want to become partners with them in sponsoring a life skills training program.

Strategy 3: Provide a Variety of Youth Activities, Programs

Young people need to be involved in stimulating, challenging and constructive youth activities which address a diversity of young people's interests and needs. Programs and activities which engage youth in contributing to the community, where they can learn new skills and values, and put their faith into action should be high on the list of every church's youth ministry. Programs and activities need to address the developmental needs of young and older adolescents and consciously promote the internal assets of youth. This does not mean that more programs will necessarily mean better programs. Youth ministries will need to be more focused so that the programs and activities they do sponsor effectively address positive youth development.

Of particular concern should be the catechetical or religious education programs. These programs should be focused on teaching knowledge of the Christian tradition *and* skills for living as disciples today. Young people need to see that the Christian faith and value system is a tremendous resource for their growth and development. They need to see that the Christian faith gives meaning to their "real life" issues. We have suggested that life skills training become an integral part of religious education programming, but this emphasis on skills for Christian living needs to go further. They need to develop practical skills for living the Christian faith in the world today. This style of religious education also encourages independent thinking and questioning and effectively helps youth to apply their faith to daily decisions and life experiences.

Strategy 4: Provide Meaningful Service Involvement

Service is an excellent way to develop prosocial (caring) values and behaviors in young people and to promote their faith growth. Every youth ministry should include a well organized community service component. Be sure to include education, action, and reflection, as well as a wide variety of service options to respond to the diversity of youth interests.

You may want to explore the possibilities of incorporating a youth component into parish service projects by identifying which parish groups are engaged in service to the community and then working with them to include youth in their present and future service projects. Another way to utilize existing service programming is to invite the young people to sponsor or adopt a local, diocesan or national service project and invite other youth, and/or families and/or the entire parish community to participate with them in the action. By taking leadership for service, young people can be the catalysts for involving the entire parish community in service. Projects like *Operation Rice Bowl* from Catholic Relief Services or *CROP Walk* from Church World Service are examples of pre-designed national projects.

Strategy 5: Engage Youth in Leadership Positions, Training

We promote positive youth development when we provide youth the opportunities to engage in leadership *and* the knowledge and skills needed for effective leadership. Nothing builds more involvement and ownership than engaging young people in leadership roles in the school, youth programming, and/or the parish community. This is a great way to build mentoring relationships between adults and youth, and to utilize the gifts, talents, and energy of youth in the parish community. Think about all possibilities for leadership in your current youth ministry and in the ministries, programs, and activities of the parish — parish council, parish committees (liturgy, social activities, religious education), parish social events, children's religious education. Be sure to provide leadership training for youth so that they can succeed in their new roles.

Strategy 6: Address Specific At-Risk Concerns Among Youth

Provide information and educational programs about issues such as sexuality and substance abuse *and* connect these issues to their faith, values, and experiences of the Christian faith community. A variety of excellent program resources are available for your use. Many communities have resource people who conduct programs on these topics that could be utilized in your programming. Once again, investigate what other churches, schools and other youth organizations in the community are already doing. You might want to partner with them in sponsoring programs on at-risk issues.

Strategy 7: Create Opportunities for Youth to Contribute to the Church Community

Young people need to feel valued and accepted by the community. They need to know that there are meaningful roles for them within the life of the community which provide experiences of *real* responsibility. We are all too familiar with examples of "token" roles for youth in church life. When young people realize they have no voice or responsibility, their disappointment and disenchantment with church runs very deep. Youth need to be able to participate in meaningful, valued activities and roles in the Christian community. Involvement in parish ministries and leadership roles enhances their sense of responsibility and purpose and nurtures a sense of belonging and loyalty to the community. Through meaningful participation young people can learn the story of our faith experientially. They have the opportunity to develop intergenerational relationships which are so important for sharing faith and promoting growth.

Meaningful involvement of young people is the responsibility of the entire community. Leaders in ministry with youth have a special role in advocating for youth participation and in becoming the catalysts for creating new opportunities for youth in the community. Leaders will need to complement their youth-focused programming with community-based programming. This may mean reducing youth-only programming so that time and resources can be allocated to community opportunities. We have already mentioned several strategies you can use to create opportunities for youth to become contributing members, such as leadership and service.

The liturgical life of the parish offers another opportunity by involving youth in liturgical ministries, such as lectors, greeters (hospitality ministry), and music ministers (voice or instruments). First, identify youth who are good singers or instrumentalists (check out the school band and choir) and get them involved in music ministry. Identify artists and encourage them to use their gifts in planning the environment for the various liturgical seasons. Establish an apprenticeship program and/or specific liturgical and skill training for youth involved in liturgical ministries. A second approach is to involve youth in the preparation and leadership of seasonal (Advent/Christmas, Lent/Easter, Pentecost) or ethnic celebrations. For example, young people with dramatic and musical talent can take responsibility for a "Living" Stations of the Cross during Holy Week. Another way to do this is to involve youth in the preparation and leadership of special youth Eucharistic liturgies (e.g., back-to-school liturgy, graduation liturgy), prayer services or communal reconciliation services.

Strategy 8: Provide Caring and Supportive Relationships

Every adolescent needs at least one caring, consistent adult in his or her life beyond their parents. Youth need more meaningful contact with adults who they can have frequent, in-depth conversations and go to for advice and support. Every church community and its youth ministry can nurture caring and supportive relationships through mentoring, youth-to-youth peer ministry, and intergenerational programming.

Mentoring is a ideal way to promote positive youth development. Five elements are important in mentor relationships:

- The adult takes a personal interest in the particular young person. The adolescent comes to feel a sense of personal worthiness just from seeing his or her particular and unique worth reflected in the eyes of an adult who is not a parent.

- The adult tends to become a model for the young person. The adolescent sees in the adult the beliefs, attitudes, the values, the patterns of behavior, the accomplishments, and the style of life that, to a significant degree, the adolescent desires to emulate and adopt as his or her own. The adult's response is to become teacher, guide, counselor, sponsor, and host to the young person.

- The adult acts as a guarantor for the adolescent. He or she lets the young person know that in experiences of struggle, doubt, and confusion or during feelings of inadequacy about the journey ahead, the young person is not alone. Others have been there before, have found resources within themselves that they did not know were there, and made it.

- The adult provides an open ear to the adolescent.

- The adult sometimes take on the role of advocate. As an advocate, the adult will stand up for the adolescent when the young person comes up against destructive opposition. In short, the adult empowers the young person when the adolescent's own power is not enough (Dykstra).

Potential strategies for intentionally creating mentor relationships include a matchmaker program between youth and adults who have similar interests, vocational counseling programs with a one-on-one relationship between an adult in a career and a young person exploring that career, one-on-one teaching, apprenticeships between adult leaders in parish ministries and committees and youth who want to be leaders in these areas, and youth programs which invite adults from the community to participate.

Strategy 9: Partner with Parents and Families

Families and churches share the task of promoting healthy growth. Youth ministry must work to establish a partnership with families in this common task. This means creating a family perspective in youth ministry and church life. Creating a family perspective can take many forms:

- **Incorporating a family perspective and family involvement into current programming.** This involves examining our current youth ministry efforts and bringing family concerns into youth programming, connecting with the realities of family life, applying the learnings from a youth program into family life, and/or designing activities that encourage young people to consult with and learning from the experience of family members. It may mean transforming youth-only programming into parent-youth programming by incorporating a parent component into a program or by adding a parallel program for parents with similar topics and time schedule as the youth program. Other ways to develop a family perspective include keeping families informed of activities, giving them opportunities to consult in the planning process, and inviting family members to contribute their time and energies to the youth ministry effort through a family advisory board and through volunteer leadership roles.

  Church-wide intergenerational and/or family programming also has many benefits for youth. Explore the possibilities of designing or redesigning existing church programming with a family or intergenerational focus, e.g., socials, picnics, worship experiences, religious education programs, parish mission, Advent programming, Lenten programming, ethnic events and celebrations.

- **Creating in-home resources and activities.** Helping families grow in faith and build stronger relationships is the goal of in-home resources and activities. This can take a variety of forms such as providing parenting resources (print or video), family rituals and celebrations, (e.g., a family reconciliation service), and family activity suggestions. Many current youth and adult programs can be redesigned to include a take-home resource or activity for the family. Newsletters can become an excellent vehicle for communicating in-home activities and parenting suggestions. Remember that families need to experience the support of the church community as they seek to share faith and values at home.

• **Developing a Resource Center**. Giving parents and family members access to quality print, video, and community resources is the goal of a resource center. A resource center becomes an information clearinghouse and rental library for families and leaders. The center would contain resources (books, videos, pamphlets) on parenting, improving family relationships, family activities, community resources (counseling services), etc.

Strategy 10: Provide Parent Education, Encouragement, Support Networks, and Resources

Parent education is one of the best investments youth ministry leaders can make in the positive development of youth. Many current research studies point to the need for building the competence and confidence of parents through parent education training and resources. Providing parents with developmentally appropriate knowledge and skills for parenting adolescents through workshops, courses, and resources, building support networks among parents, and making available in-home parenting resources (print, video, cassettes, etc.) are three strategies for strengthening the skills of parents. Parent-youth programming can feel overwhelming so you may want to utilize guest speakers, video-based programs, or packaged programs from the diocese or other agencies. Parishes can provide an important service to parents and the community by placing a priority on providing organized, systematic parent education, and by intentionally creating support groups and networks for parents.

Strategy 11: Provide Culturally Relevant Programming

We have already seen that an important developmental need of minority youth is to provide them with opportunities to achieve a positive orientation toward mainstream American culture and their own culture and to affirm their ethnicity through observation of ceremonies, retention of native language, and reinforcement of specific attitudes, beliefs, and practices. A fully multicultural approach to positive youth development views ethnicity and culture as core features of identity and behavior, and it emphasizes pluralism in all aspects of organizational life. This approach stresses that mainstream American culture is one of many as it attempts to draw on the strengths of other cultural systems for its goals as well as its operations. In this model, all youth are made to feel welcome and empowered; leaders reflect the ethnocultural characteristics of the programs' participants; all staff are trained to be culturally competent; program participants and their families are equitably represented on advisory councils; and program content is culturally appropriate and relevant to the needs of participants.

Churches should recognize that the specific content of adolescent tasks and competencies varies by culture. For example, although the attainment of individual autonomy constitutes a universal task of adolescence, the specific meaning of autonomy is constructed differently across cultural groups. Similarly, conceptions of proper social relationships vary. Dating and socializing with friends outside of the home may be considered appropriate adolescent behaviors among Americans, but are viewed as inappropriate among many recently arrived Southeast Asian families. Youth programs that ignore such realities risk being unsuccessful with some populations.

Youth ministry programming can help young people learn about, understand, and appreciate people with backgrounds different from their own. Even churches that are located in homogeneous communities, with no significant number of potential minority participants, can design programs that convey the value of diversity and that create opportunities for multicultural awareness and appreciation. Youth programs can also counteract prejudice, racism, and discrimination. They can teach by example — by becoming themselves models of fairness and nondiscrimination. They can also diminish racism's harmful consequences. Explicit programs in racism and oppression awareness can assist all youth in developing effective communication skills in a multicultural context and minority youth in developing skills for coping with and overcoming social barriers to minority achievement. Such programs can benefit not only minority teens but also those from majority groups by helping both groups realize the nature and extent of racism.

Youth ministries should purposefully create environments that not only meet psychosocial needs and develop competencies but also celebrate and build on aspects of participants' racial and ethnic backgrounds in the process. Adolescents are poised to take risks, to widen their circle of relationships and affiliations, and to explore actively their worlds and themselves (*A Matter of Time* 83-85).

Strategy 12: Get Involved in Community Networking

Churches need to work with other community organizations in a common effort to promote healthy adolescent development. Sharing resources, co-sponsoring programming, mobilizing the community to address youth issues are only some of the ways churches and community organizations can work together for the common good of all young people.

One idea for using community resources within youth ministry is to develop and distribute a directory of recommended counseling resources that youth and their families can use for assistance in times of trouble. A parish or school can print cards with phone numbers of crisis intervention services, support groups, resource people and agencies. The directory can also include a list of community educational programs and resources (books and videos) for youth and/or parents that address adolescent/family concerns and problems. A second approach is to create a calendar that lists all of the *recommended* parish and community events for youth and for families in a given month or season (3-4 months). This is a great way to alert youth and their families to upcoming programs, activities, and events and to invite them to participate. Make sure that the calendar includes pertinent information on each event. Mail the calendar to every youth and their parents or insert it into the parish bulletin. Be sure to highlight parish activities.

One way to begin collaborating with other faith institutions, schools, and community organizations is by convening a *Community Forum* of leaders. The initial purpose of the Community Forum is to build relationships among leaders, to share information about each organization's approach to youth development (programs, resources), and to begin the process of building a comprehensive, communitywide approach to positive youth development. Such sharing can begin to produce the common ground for building partnerships and sharing programs and resources. A Community Forum can lead toward the creation of a community-wide vision for positive youth development. Further along it might lead toward a detailed action plan to promote positive youth development with an emphasis on increasing youth access to effective schools, families and youth-serving organizations. The gathering of leaders could also provide impetus for advocacy efforts to obtain greater state or federal or foundation support for school effectiveness, parent education, after school care, prevention programming, and other efforts crucial for promoting positive youth development.

CONCLUSION

In *A Matter of Time* the Carnegie Council on Adolescent Development identifies 10 principles that should guide our programming as we seek to implement the strategies and create a comprehensive approach to positive youth development. Responsive proactive community programs for adolescents should:

• tailor their content and processes to the needs and interests of adolescents

- recognize, value, and respond to the diverse backgrounds and experiences that exist among adolescents

- work collectively as well as individually to extend their reach to underserved adolescents

- compete actively for adolescents' time and attention

- strengthen the quality and diversity of their adult leadership

- reach out to families, schools, and other community partners in youth development

- enhance the role of young people as resources to their community

- serve as vigorous advocates for and with youth

- specify and evaluate their intended outcomes

- establish solid organizational structures, including energetic and committed board leadership (*A Matter of Time* 79).

Now it is time to begin. It is time to evaluate efforts, to build on strengths and identify areas of need, and to develop those strategies that will promote positive youth development in more effective, comprehensive ways. The essays and resources offered in Section III of this book and in its *Activity Manual* are designed to assist you in your work. The challenges and opportunities await!

TABLE 1: THE CHANGES OF EARLY ADOLESCENCE

Physical Development
- developing secondary sex characteristics and the capacity to reproduce
- growing stronger and taller
- being sensitive about physical changes and confused about their emerging sexuality
- incorporating their bodily changes into their own self image as male or female

Intellectual Development
- beginning to move from concrete thinking (what is) to abstract thinking, "formal operations," (what might be true if...)
- questioning and testing adults' statements and evaluating adults' values
- being painfully self-conscious and critical, idealistic, argumentative, self-centered
- expanding interests; intense, short term enthusiasm

Identity Development
- requiring time to reflect upon the new reactions they receive from others and to construct a consistent self-image from the many different mirrors in which they view themselves
- discovering who they are as unique persons with abilities, interests and goals
- seeking limited independence and autonomy from parents and adults

Moral Development
- engaging in more complex decision-making process
- resolving moral dilemmas in terms of the expectations of someone or something other than themselves, which can be (a) family, friends or other significant persons or (b) what the law or the system of good order calls for in a given situation

Interpersonal Development
- relying on parents and families in setting values and giving affection
- identifying more strongly with the peer group for belonging and deepening friendships
- entering a broader social world of middle school, peer groups, and activity groups
- developing the ability to consider the feelings, actions, and needs of those within a relationship
- learning how to relate to the opposite sex (what to say and how to behave)

Faith Development
- deriving their faith from parents and family through earlier identification and modeling
- developing their faith and identity, establishing a set of religious beliefs, attitudes and values, through the experiences of participation and belonging in a caring faith community where they are valued

TABLE 2: THE CHANGES OF OLDER ADOLESCENCE

Intellectual Development
- dealing with more complex intellectual challenges
- developing the ability to engage in reflective thinking ("what do I think?" and "why do I think that?"), i.e., the ability to think about what they know, value, and believe, thereby making it possible for them to grow toward a personal identity, a personal moral value system, and a personal faith
- thinking about and planning for the future

Identity Development
- beginning the process of establishing a personal identity, a meaningful self-concept, which includes an acceptance of one's sexuality, a sex-role identity (self-definition as a man or woman), decision-making regarding education or career choice, and a commitment to a personally-held system of values, religious beliefs, vocational goals, and philosophy of life
- shifting from inherited authority (especially the family) to self-chosen authority (eventually oneself), often by establishing a relational identity that is powerfully shaped by significant others (peers and adults)
- experiencing a period of questioning, reevaluation, and experimentation as they seek to develop a unified, consistent self-concept
- developing increasing autonomy in making personal decisions, assuming responsibility for oneself, and regulating one's own behavior

Moral Development
- exercising moral judgments in matters of much greater complexity as they seek to establish a more personal form of moral reasoning
- reevaluating the moral values received from family, church, and significant others (adults, peers)
- searching for a moral code which preserves their personal integrity and provides the basis for developing an internalized moral value system that can guide their behavior

Interpersonal Development
- moving toward greater personal intimacy and adult sexuality
- developing the capability for more mutual, trusting, deep, and enduring personal friendships with members of the same sex and opposite sex that provide acceptance, love, affirmation for self-image, and the opportunity to honestly share their deepest selves
- expanding their perspective to encompass the larger world by seeking to comprehend more deeply the motives, feelings, and thought patterns of individuals and groups of peoples outside their personal experience

Faith Development
- exploring and questioning the faith handed down by family and church as they search for a style of faith and belief which is more personal to oneself
- beginning the process of taking responsibility for one's own faith life, commitments, lifestyle, beliefs and attitudes
- exploring a personal relationship with God who knows, accepts and confirms them deeply, and with Jesus Christ through his teaching, example, and presence in one's life

End Notes

[1] *Beyond Rhetoric — A New American Agenda for Children and Families*. Final Report of the National Commission on Children. Washington, DC: National Commission on Children, 1991.

[2] *The Troubled Journey* study reports on more than 46,000 young Americans in grades 6 through 12 and yields information of great significance to all those who are interested in providing youth with a chance to grow up healthy. The students included in this research come mainly from the Midwest; most of them live in communities under 100,000 in population. Ninety percent of them are white. However, in spite of this sample, on key indicators for which representative national data are available (e.g., alcohol use, tobacco use, sexual abuse, involvement in extracurricular activities, and exposure to television), percentages in this study are remarkably similar to those of national data on in-school youth. Material in this essay is drawn from *Source* 6.3 (December 1990) and *Source* 7.1 (April 1991) published by the Search Institute, 122 W. Franklin, Suite 525, Minneapolis, MN 55404. Additional material is drawn from *The Troubled Journey: A Profile of American Youth* developed by Peter Benson of the Search Institute and published by RESPECTEEN, Lutheran Brotherhood, Minneapolis, MN 55415. You can order an overview of *The Troubled Journey* by calling 1-800-888-3820. You can have this survey administered in your school system. It is available through RESPECTEEN at no charge and will highlight important issues for community discussion and action. There is no better way to raise the community's consciousness about youth than through current information about your community's own youth.

[3] Some of the material for the development changes and developmental needs of young adolescents is drawn from the following sources: *A Portrait of Young Adolescents in the 1990s* by Peter Scales (Carrboro, NC: Center for Early Adolescence, 1991), *Director's Manual for the Discovering Program* by Michael Carotta (Winona, MN: St. Mary's Press, 1989), and *Access Guides to Youth Ministry: Early Adolescent Ministry* edited by John Roberto (New Rochelle, NY: Don Bosco Multimedia, 1991).

[4] Some of the material for the development changes and developmental needs of older adolescents is drawn from *Adolescent Spirituality* by Charles Shelton (Chicago: Loyola University Press, 1983).

[5] Material in this section is drawn from "Backbone: Essential for Survival on the Troubled Journey" *Source* 7.1 (April 1991).

[6] Material in this section is drawn from "The Troubled Journey: New Light on Growing Up Healthy" *Source* 6.3 (December 1990).

Works Cited

A Matter of Time. Carnegie Council on Adolescent Development. New York: Carnegie Corporation of New York, 1993.

"Backbone: Essential for Survival on the Troubled Journey." *Source* 7.1 (April 1991).

Benson, Peter. *The Troubled Journey: A Profile of American Youth*. Minneapolis, MN: RESPECTEEN, Lutheran Brotherhood, 1991.

Dykstra, Craig. "Agenda for Youth Ministry: Problems, Questions, and Strategies." *Readings and Resources in Youth Ministry*. Ed. Michael Warren. Winona, MN: St. Mary's Press, 1987.

Roberto, John, Editor. *Access Guides to Youth Ministry: Early Adolescent Ministry*. New Rochelle, NY: Don Bosco Multimedia, 1991.

Scales, Peter. *A Portrait of Young Adolescents in the 1990s*. Carrboro, NC: Center for Early Adolescence, 1991.

"The Troubled Journey: New Light on Growing Up Healthy." *Source* 6.3 (December

1990).

Williams, Dorothy. "Religion in Adolescence: Dying, Dormant, or Developing." *SOURCE* 5.4 (December 1989).

CHAPTER 3

THE NATURE AND SCOPE OF ADOLESCENT PROBLEMS

David A. Hamburg

THE EVOLUTION OF ADOLESCENCE

From time to time, we read about the death of an adolescent who was at the peak of youthful energy and promise, with the prospect of a long life in view. All these accounts are shocking, yet we become inured to them because they come along so frequently. The dramatic instances of adolescent suicide, homicide, drinking and driving, or drug overdose highlight the general predicament of adolescent development in a time of world transformation. How can a person with so much potential to build a rewarding and constructive life snuff it out so casually?

It is useful to view adolescence in a historical and even an evolutionary perspective. Adolescence is a time when our children experience drastic changes, both physical and behavioral. The timing of puberty is controlled by the brain, which stimulates the secretion of sex hormones, a development that evolved over millions of years. Our gradual understanding of this ancient biological system has made puberty one of the frontiers of neuroendocrine research — the interplay of brain and hormones. It is now also becoming a frontier of the behavioral sciences.

While the structure of our biological machinery has a genetic basis, its operation is linked to our environment. Drastic changes in the social and economic fabric of our lives since the Industrial Revolution have affected not only the timing of puberty but the whole nature of the adolescent experience. Today's adolescents undergo their transition from childhood to adulthood in circumstances that are unique in the long history of our species.

One important change — in fact, a distinctly human evolutionary novelty — is the lengthy period of adolescence. We now have two largely separate crucial periods in the transition from childhood to adulthood. At the beginning of adolescence, our children undergo a biological change; at the end of adolescence, a psychosocial change. For reasons not fully understood but including better nutrition and fewer serious infections, adolescence now starts earlier than it used to and ends later. The onset of menstruation, on average, occurs at twelve and a half years in the United States, whereas 150 years ago the average age at menarche was sixteen. In less-developed countries, the age of menarche is still high, but it is decreasing. Boys are also reaching reproductive maturity at an earlier age. Reproductively mature persons now spend years in childlike roles, or in any case in nonadult status, most of them for a decade or more — especially if they pursue higher education. The end of adolescence is ambiguous. When is a person considered fully adult in modern circumstances? How does the modern adolescent adapt to the lengthy transition?

By and large, it is not until roughly the end of the teen years that adolescents reach a fully adult state in brain development, let alone social maturity. The biological, cognitive, psychological, and social differences between the eleven-year-old and the nineteen-year-old are so great that it is barely meaningful to cover both under the label "adolescence." Yet most adolescents are ten to fifteen years old when they are exposed to sexuality, alcohol and other drugs, smoking, and the temptation to engage in a variety of health-damaging behaviors.

Complicating adolescence today is the easy availability of high-risk activities or substances that adolescents generally view as recreational, tension-relieving, and gratifying. Adolescents have ready access to deadly poison in the guise of casual experience: drugs, vehicles, weapons, and the many ways in which one's body may be used dangerously.

Exploratory behavior is central to early adolescence. But a large proportion of early adolescents are not well prepared to make informed decisions about the risks and opportunities they encounter. In many ways, they resemble a larger version of toddlers — having the newly acquired capacity to get into all sorts of novel and risky situations, but all too little judgment and information on which to base decisions about how to handle themselves. Historically, much of the information and worldview was shaped by the nuclear and extended family: parents, older siblings, older peers, and various other relatives. Today, adolescents' information comes largely from the media and unrelated peers, and much of it clashes with parental expectations.

A third historic change is the difficulty adolescents now have foreseeing the years ahead. In premodern times, children were regarded as small, inexperienced adults whose sole task was preparation for adult life. They had abundant opportunity to observe and imitate their parents and other adults performing the roles that they would one day occupy. Career options were limited. Strong social-support networks provided predictability, guidance, and strong coping resources in established, small societies. In today's highly technological and rapidly changing world, such direct modeling is much less widely available. Most societies are too large and their economies too complex to permit children and adolescents much direct observation of adult roles, especially occupational ones. Many jobs change so fast that skills needed today are obsolete fifteen years from now. Moreover, traditional social-support networks have been disrupted. Science and technology have liberated adolescents from the drudgery experienced by their predecessors but, as a paradox of success, have made it harder for them to view the future. What is the adult world, anyway? Is it really what you see on television?

Most early adolescents yearn to be adults without actually understanding what adults do and are. Thus, one of the most important things we can do for adolescents is give them a clearer view of constructive adult roles and what it means to be a respected adult.

One of the key tasks of later adolescence is to move toward a career that can earn respect and be compatible with one's sense of personal worth. We therefore need to ask what various institutions — particularly schools — can do to help adolescents build those careers.

Despite so much change in circumstances, the fundamental tasks of growing up endure:

- to find a place in a valued group that gives a sense of belonging;

- to identify and master tasks that are generally recognized as having value and therefore earn respect by acquiring the skill to cope with them;

- to acquire a sense of worth as a person;

- to develop reliable and predictable relationships with other people, especially a few close friends and loved ones.

The growing adolescent has several specific developmental tasks:

- Moving toward independence from parents, siblings, and childhood friends while retaining significant and enduring ties;

- Developing increasing autonomy in making personal decisions, assuming responsibility for oneself, and regulating one's own behavior;

- Establishing new friendships;

- Moving toward greater personal intimacy and adult sexuality;

- Dealing with more complex intellectual challenges.

These are steps every adolescent must take on the road to adulthood, yet major indicators show that in contemporary society large numbers of adolescents cannot find avenues through which to accomplish them. The swiftness, in historical terms, of these drastic changes has outrun our understanding and institutional capacity to adapt. We urgently need to improve our capabilities to deal with the challenges of adolescent development. We may need to bring about a sea of change in adolescent's preparation for adult life, taking into account the drastic world transformation that has recently occurred and is still rapidly under way.

The Burden of Illness, Ignorance, and Wasted Potential

Although most children grow up to be healthy and whole adults, substantial numbers encounter serious problems along the way that threaten their survival or leave their entire lives warped or unfulfilled. Some children are at great risk from the moment of birth, or even before; others are most vulnerable during early adolescence. The physical, social, and emotional changes of adolescence intersect with the new intellectual tasks and organizational structure in the middle-grade school. (This term covers both the junior-high schools and the middle schools. These overlap greatly and, taken together, they constitute the special institution we have created for education in early adolescence). For many students, the emerging sense of one's own future may be bleak, especially in areas of high joblessness, poverty, and disintegrated communities. During adolescence, a significant number of young people from many social groups drop out of school, commit violence or otherwise criminal acts, become pregnant, become mentally ill, abuse drugs or alcohol, attempt suicide, die, or are disabled from injuries.

In early adolescence, millions of American youths are at risk of reaching adulthood unable to sustain jobs, deep commitments in human relationships, or the responsibilities of participation in a democratic society. They often suffer from unrealized intellectual potential, indifference to good health, and cynicism about humane values.

These adolescents — like many others — are sorely tempted and often pressured to use alcohol, cigarettes, and illicit drugs. Far too many live in neighborhoods so dangerous that they fear walking to school. Many consider sexual experience at this age to be almost obligatory — a far cry from their parents' experience; they are prompted to some degree by incessant stimulation in movies, television, and music. Adolescents are similarly bombarded with messages about big money and conspicuous success as putative badges of real adulthood. At the same time they are exposed to messages of concern for others, helping, even sacrifice for the common good. These conflicting messages are not easy to reconcile.

Stable, close-knit communities where people know each other well and maintain a strong ethic of mutual aid are less common than they were a generation or two ago. The nature of the economy has changed so rapidly that unskilled youth can find only low-paying work, often with little prospect of future improvement. Entire industries have virtually disappeared in recent years. Economic opportunities of adulthood are obscure to most adolescents. In this time of drastic change, young people need informed adult guidance from parents and others. Yet parents often mistake the stirring of independent thinking for the capacity to make informed, mature decisions. Adolescents do indeed have a growing desire for autonomy but also a continuing need for support, encouragement, and guidance. They need help making the developmental transition for dependency to interdependency with parents, friends, relatives, and other adults. Although they are renegotiating relationships with adults, and especially parents, in ways that are often tense and occasionally hostile, adolescents typically wish to maintain ties with and continue to receive help from the adults in their lives.

Let us now take a closer look at the common pitfalls today's adolescents face.

Substance Abuse

Experimentation with drugs, cigarettes, and alcohol is quite common during adolescence. The annual survey of the National Institute on Drug Abuse showed that most of the high-school class of 1987 (92%) had used alcohol at some time. Sixty-seven percent has smoked cigarettes, 50% had used marijuana, 22% has used stimulants, 15% had used cocaine, and 6% had used crack. Males had higher rates of use than females for most of these substances.

Far fewer adolescents use drugs, cigarettes, and alcohol habitually than have ever tried them. Among the high-school class of 1987, 5% had drunk alcohol daily during the month before they were surveyed, 19% had smoked cigarettes daily, and 3% had used marijuana daily. Binge drinking, on the other hand, is relatively common: 37% of high-school seniors (29% of females and 46% of males) reported having had five or more drinks in a row during the prior two weeks.

Smoking, drinking, and drug use frequently begin in early adolescence. For example, over half of those who smoke in the twelfth grade began daily cigarette smoking before tenth grade. Three out of five high-school seniors who have ever used alcohol, and about half of those who have ever used marijuana, first used it before tenth grade. Similar statistics apply to nearly all other drugs, except for cocaine, which was rarely used before high school for the class of 1987 — though its use in early adolescence has increased since then.

Alcohol is frequently involved in motor-vehicle accidents. In approximately half the motor-vehicle fatalities involving an adolescent driver, the driver has an elevated blood alcohol level. Alcohol is also frequently implicated when adolescents die as pedestrians or while using recreational vehicles. Injuries resulting from accidents account for the largest number of hospital stays among twelve- to seventeen-year-olds. The combination of driving and drinking does not affect only those adolescents who are old enough to drive. Nearly one-third of eighth-grade students report having ridden in a car during the previous month with a driver under the influence of alcohol.

Alcohol use has become a more serious problem among ten- to fifteen-year-olds over the past two decades. Drinking patterns have changed remarkably. A greater proportion of early adolescents drink alcoholic beverages, have their first drinking experience earlier, and report more frequent intoxication. Although girls drink less than boys, the portion who drink and who report intoxication has increased more rapidly for girls than for boys. There are similar patterns of increase in cigarette smoking among girls, and the gender gap in the use of illegal drugs has narrowed in the past ten years.

A striking increase in marijuana use began in the second half of the sixties, but has leveled off in recent years. Still, more than half of high-school seniors have had some experience with the drug, and the decline in marijuana use halted in 1985. Among dropouts, its use is at higher levels than among those in school. Between 1975 and 1980 there was a significant increase in first use of marijuana in early adolescents and that has been a common pattern ever since. Early use of marijuana has been shown to be associated with higher likelihood of using more dangerous drugs later.

Drugs that are manufactured or sold outside the law often are contaminated, of variable and unpredictable potency, or misrepresented — all factors associated with a higher incidence of medical emergencies. Moreover, the use of two or more illegal drugs — often along with alcohol — increases one's health risks considerably.

During the past decade, cocaine has emerged from the shadows as a major public-health threat. Epidemiologic surveys and public-health surveillance systems have documented remarkable increases in cocaine use not only in the general adult population but also among high-school students. As the use of cocaine has increased, particularly with the introduction of the inexpensive form of crack, so too have emergency-room visits, overdose deaths, and medical problems reflected by more and more adolescents entering treatment. The prevalence of "standard" cocaine use in the general population has leveled off since 1979, but the adverse consequences have continued to increase sharply. While there was some evidence that cocaine use reached a plateau in 1990, the problem is complicated by increased combination-drug use and by a shift to more dangerous ways of taking the drug.

Sexuality, Pregnancy, and Disease

The earlier onset of puberty is lengthening the period during which adolescents' physical maturity exceeds their emotional and cognitive maturity. Early initiation of sexual activity puts adolescents at risk of sexually transmitted diseases and unplanned parenthood. A recent survey found that by age fifteen, 13% of white males and 6% of white females had had sexual intercourse, 45% of black males and 10% of black females had had intercourse. By age seventeen, 44% of white males, 28% of white females, 82% of black males, and 45% of black females had had intercourse. Sexual activity is more common among adolescents who attend high schools with high dropout rates or who have poorly educated mothers.

Among sexually active girls aged fifteen to nineteen in 1982, about 15% had never used contraception. Over half had not used contraception when they first had intercourse. Black adolescents and younger adolescents generally were less likely than other adolescents to have used contraception.

Sexually active adolescents have much higher rates of gonorrhea, syphilis, and pelvic inflammatory disease than do older groups. An estimated one-quarter of sexually active adolescents are infected with a sexually transmitted disease before graduating from high school. In recent years, the AIDS epidemic has powerfully complicated this problem.

In 1986 there were about a million pregnancies among girls under twenty, of which about half resulted in births. Most of these pregnancies were unintended. Eighteen- to nineteen-year-olds accounted for nearly two-thirds of the births, but 180,000 births were to girls aged seventeen or younger and 10,000 were to girls aged fourteen and younger. Early motherhood is associated with dropping out of high school, low skills, and poverty.

While the overall rate of births to adolescents has fallen in the last few decades, the average age of initiation of sexual activity has decreased, the birthrate for those under fifteen has increased, and an increasing proportion of adolescent births are out of wedlock. During the past decade, research has clarified the medical, personal, social, and economic consequences of these early pregnancy and childbearing patterns. The consequences of pregnancy for an eighteen- or nineteen-year-old are very different from the consequences for someone still of school age, particularly if the girl is under fifteen years old. The consequences of school-age childbearing are almost all damaging — for the mother, the father, the child, and society. Therefore, a focus on early-adolescent pregnancy — as well as other *early*-adolescent problems — is crucial.

In the United States, the women at highest risk are very young, black, marginally nourished, and from a low socioeconomic status; they do not seek prenatal care. Research findings are strong on the damaging outcomes of early-adolescent pregnancy. Biologic risks to the mother include toxemia of pregnancy and complications during labor and delivery. Socioeconomic risks include interruption of the mother's education, which in turn fosters poor occupational prospects and an increased probability of a lifetime of poverty and less ability to provide a healthy environment for the baby. Infants of young adolescent mothers also are at health risk, especially if their mothers are regular smokers or users of alcohol or other drugs. They are likely to be born too soon or at low birth weight; this in turn predisposes them to a variety of developmental disorders carrying the risk of permanent disability.

Caretaking by very young mothers is also a problem. Adolescent mothers are often less responsible to the needs of the infant than older mothers are. They also tend to have more babies in rapid succession than do older mothers, placing their infants at greater biological and behavioral risk. Children of adolescent mothers tend to have more cognitive, emotional, behavioral, and health problems at all stages of development than do children of fully adult mothers.

The childbearing rate of American adolescents is among the highest in the technically advanced nations of the world. Adolescents account for two thirds of all out-of-wedlock births. Although birthrates among both older adolescents and adults have declined since 1970, the birthrate among girls under fifteen has not. There are 1.3 million children now living with teenage mothers, about half of whom are married. An additional 6 million children under age five are living with mothers who were adolescents when they gave birth.

The majority of adolescent mothers drop out of school. Early childbearing is a route into poverty and a major obstacle to breaking out of intergenerational poverty. The outlook for the infant is often bleak. When the adolescent's extended family offers child-rearing support, the child's prospects improve. And if the adolescent girl has only one child, the outlook is more hopeful for both.

Social isolation and other socioeconomic stresses adversely affect very young fathers as well as mothers. The adolescent father is launched on a downward trajectory similar to that shown in studies of adolescent mothers — low educational accomplishment and employment opportunities, poverty, early divorce, and frequent changes of martial partner.

Throughout most of human history, adolescent childbearing — within four years of menarche, while the mother was in her late teens — was common. But in those societies the community provided relatively stable employment and predictable networks of social support and cultural guidance for the young parents. For such adolescents to set up a household apart from either family was rare in preindustrial societies. Even more rare was the single-parent family, and rarest of all was a socially isolated, very young mother largely lacking an effective network of social support. Today these conditions are common.

Nutrition, Activity, and Fitness

The adolescent fondness for junk foods and fad diets contributes to their inadequate or poor nutrition. The National Health and Nutrition Examination Survey documented the tendency of adolescents both below and above the poverty level to take in less than the recommended daily allowance of calories and iron. On the other hand, about 10% of adolescents take in far too many calories and become obese. A common form of adolescent obesity is the consequence of chronic overeating because of depression, passivity, and low self-esteem. If this dietary pattern becomes firmly established, it can lead to cardiovascular disease, diabetes, and other health problems over the long term.

One in two hundred twelve- to eighteen-year-old females develop anorexia nervosa, a self-starvation through fanatical dieting. Somewhat more common is bulimia, a binge-and-purge pattern of behavior. Both bulimia and anorexia nervosa are associated with serious medical complications.

Physical inactivity is much more widespread among young people than it was a few decades ago. A sizable minority of ten- to seventeen-year-olds are weak or uncoordinated enough to be classified as physically underdeveloped by the standards of the President's Council on Physical Fitness and Sports. Here again, if the tentative patterns of adolescence become crystallized in a long-term pattern of behavior, these individuals put themselves at risk for cardiovascular disease, pulmonary difficulty, and lack of physical vigor in the adult years.

Depression and Suicide

Mood fluctuation and transient depression are common among adolescents. The hormonal and neuroendocrine changes of puberty along with major changes in the social environment and stressful life transitions, all contribute to the problem. One national survey found mild depressive symptoms in 34% of males and 15% of female adolescents. In another sample, 6% had clinically significant depressive symptoms.

For some adolescents, depression is a precursor of suicide or attempted suicide. Suicide accounts for 6% of deaths among ten- to fourteen-year-olds, and 12% of deaths among fifteen- to nineteen-year-olds. It is more common among males than females, and more common among whites than blacks.

In addition to suffering depression, many adolescents feel driven to suicide by some combination of substance abuse, trouble with the law, intense anxiety in the face of social or academic challenges, feeling of personal worthlessness, impulsivity, guilt, and shame. Some suicide victims end their lives after a pattern of destructiveness to others, highlighting a link between suicide and violence.

Delinquency and Violence

Delinquency and antisocial behaviors are widespread, associated with but certainly not limited to conditions of poverty and educational failure. Delinquency is more frequent in adolescents from homes characterized by poor paternal supervision, extremes of discipline (absent or severe), minimal involvement by fathers in family activities, and little time spent at home. Intense family discord, both in childhood and in adolescence, is one of many factors that increase the likelihood of delinquency. But the most profound challenge lies in the "underclass." Growing up under conditions of extreme poverty, the absence of fathers, social disintegration, minimal perception of opportunity (except for the immediacy of the lucrative drug trade), and isolation from reliably nurturant human contacts puts an emerging adolescent on a very risky path indeed.

Fifty-two out of 1,000 twelve- to fifteen-year-olds annually were victims of robbery, rape, or assault during the early eighties. Among sixteen- to nineteen-year-olds, the rate of victimization was even higher, 67.8 per 1,000. These rates are about twice as high as the rate for people aged twenty and over. Victimization is more common among males than females, and among blacks than whites. This pattern is demonstrated by the rates of homicide among these four groups. In 1985, 8.6 fifteen- to nineteen-year-olds per 100,000 were murdered. The rate for white families was 2.7 per 100,000, for nonwhite females 9.4, for white males 7.3, and for nonwhite males a remarkable 39.9 per 100,000.

Many of the perpetrators of violent crimes are also adolescents and young adults. Risk factors for serious violence include a family history of violence, poor family bonding, weak ties to school and other conventional institutions, personal beliefs that justify crime and violence under a wide range of circumstances, and involvement in peer groups that encourage these behaviors. The presence of weapons intensifies the seriousness of violent incidents. One recent survey found that 23% of thirteen- to sixteen-year-old males reported taking a knife to school at least once during the prior year.

Television is a pervasive presence in the lives of most American adolescents. One responsible estimate is that the average seventeen- to eighteen-year-old has spent 15,000 hours watching television, compared with 11,000 hours spent in school. Television programs often present violence and sex in an attractive way. Contraception is rarely mentioned. In effect, television provides young people with guidance about how to be sexy, but not much about how to be sexually responsible. Explicit linkage of sex and violence has increased in recent years. The vast exposure to televised violence during the years of growth and development is well known.

Some adolescents in turmoil are especially susceptible to this stimulation.

Adolescent Injury

Recent public-health research provides much information on the epidemiology and prevention of adolescent injury.

Injuries account for 57% of all deaths among ten- to fourteen-year-olds, and 79% among fifteen- to nineteen-year-olds. For every death from injury among youths aged thirteen to nineteen, there are an estimated 41 injury hospitalizations and 1,100 cases treated in emergency rooms. Death rates from injury are higher for males than females. Poverty is associated with greater risk or injury. Injury rates for Native Americans exceed those for blacks and whites by almost 100%, while Asians have the lowest rates. Homicide is more than five times as common among blacks than whites. Suicide is more common among whites than among blacks or Native Americans.

Motor vehicles account for the largest proportion of deaths from injury among adolescents. Young drivers are especially vulnerable to crashes at night and are disproportionately responsible for the death of others. They are less likely than older drivers to use seat belts.

Homicide is the leading cause of death for black males between the ages of fourteen and forty-four. The majority of adolescent homicide victims are killed by guns. Forty percent of homicide victims aged fifteen to twenty-four have positive blood alcohol levels, and 25% are legally intoxicated (that is, their blood alcohol is over .10%).

Suicide among adolescents has increased in recent decades; there has been a particularly dramatic increase in suicides among white males. It is the third leading cause of death for people between the ages of fifteen and twenty-four. About half of suicide victims aged eighteen to twenty-four have positive blood alcohol levels. Guns are used in the majority of suicide deaths among victims aged fifteen to nineteen. Intoxicated victims between the ages of fifteen and twenty-four are seven times as likely as sober victims to have used a gun.

Drowning accounts for over 1,200 deaths among ten- to nineteen-year-olds annually. Alcohol is involved in about 40% of drowning deaths.

Sports and recreational activities are leading sources of nonfatal injuries among adolescents. Football is one of the most hazardous athletic activities, with a rate of 28 injuries per 100 participants annually. Between 1973 and 1980, 260 high-school and college football players died.

Other recreational activities that contribute to adolescent injuries are bicycling and the use of all-terrain vehicles. Bicycling injuries among adolescents are most common at younger ages. Seventy percent of the 900 bicycling deaths and 550,000 bicycling injuries treated in emergency rooms each year are among riders under age fifteen. Bicycle crashes involving motor vehicles are more serious and tend to involve older youths. About 90% of bicycling fatalities involve motor vehicles, and largely result from head injuries. Only about 10% of recreational bicyclists use helmets. About two-thirds of the victims of bicycle-related brain injuries over age fourteen were intoxicated.

All-terrain vehicles can reach speeds as high as seventy miles per hour. They tend to be unstable, especially during turns. These vehicles were responsible for about 86,000 emergency-room admissions in 1985, and have caused twelve times more deaths than bicycles have. Adolescent males account for the majority of the cases; youths aged twelve to fifteen account for one-quarter of all injuries. Helmets are used by fewer than 20% of those injured, and head injuries are responsible for 70% of the deaths. Alcohol is involved in about one-third of the injuries affecting riders over age sixteen.

Altogether, adolescent injuries cause a surprising amount of suffering, impairment, even lifelong disability and death. Predisposing factors include poverty and low status; propensity for high-risk behavior; the search for new skills and adult status; the use of alcohol and other drugs; easy availability of dangerous objects, including weapons; and lack of information about actual risks and consequences. These risk factors apply to other adolescent casualties as well.

Living with Divorce, Single-Parent Families, and Stepfamilies

Divorce and births out of wedlock are increasingly common, so adolescents are more likely than ever to live with a single parent, to experience the breakup of their family, and to enter stepfamily relationships.

Among children aged between six and seventeen in 1985, 73% lived with two parents, 22% lived with their mother only, 3% lived with their father only, and 3% lived with neither parent. Among those who lived with their mother only, 10% lived with a divorced mother, 6% lived with mothers who were married but whose husbands were absent, 4% lived with mothers who had never married, and 2% lived with mothers who were widowed.

Single parenthood is especially common among blacks. In 1985, only 40% of black children aged from six to seventeen lived with 2 parents, and 50% lived with their mother only. Hispanic children's family arrangements fall between those of blacks and whites. In 1985, 66% of Hispanic children aged from six to seventeen lived with two parents, and 28% lived with their mother only.

Single-parent families are poor more often than two-parent families, for several reasons. One parent cannot earn as much as two; women, who head most single-parent families, do not earn as much as men on average; births to unmarried women are more common among women of low earning potential; and absent parents frequently fail to pay child support. One study of divorces that occurred during the seventies found that poverty rates for children rose from 12% before divorce to 27% after divorce. The 1987 poverty rate among female-headed families with children was 46%, compared with 8% among married-couple families.

In addition to having fewer financial resources, single parents may be less able to supervise their adolescent children. There is some evidence that both living in a single-parent family and having little parental supervision are associated with adolescent behaviors such as delinquency and substance abuse. Of course, some single parents do in fact maintain adequate supervision and overcome many difficulties, but on the average it tends to be a difficult situation for effective child-rearing, especially in poverty.

CLUSTERING OF RISKS AND PROBLEM BEHAVIORS

Since exploratory behavior is so characteristic of adolescents, and some of it is risky, we need to discuss the concept of risk here. The problem, of course, is that those behaviors that most adults recognize as threats to life and limb are not seen as risky to adolescents. In fact, adolescents do not generally have accurate perceptions of the probability, severity, and reversibility of the risks they take. To some degree, many adolescents find risk-taking behavior intrinsically pleasurable — a search for gratification through adventure and perhaps by beating the odds.

Adolescents put themselves in particular jeopardy because they often engage in several types of risky behavior simultaneously. Research done by Richard Jessor, director of the Institute for Behavioral Sciences at the University of Colorado, as well as epidemiological studies, indicate that problem drinkers are twice as likely as non-problem drinkers to have additional problem behaviors, a fact that obviously puts teens at risk.

A recent synthesis of research by Joy Dryfoos, a respected scholar in this field, documents the major extent to which adolescents tend to become involved in several problem behaviors at once. She identified seven major common antecedents of delinquency, substance abuse, teenage pregnancy, and school failure:

• Early initiation of any behavior predicts heavier involvement in it later, and more negative consequences.

• Doing poorly in school or expecting to do poorly in school predicts all problem behaviors.

• Impulsive behavior, truancy, and antisocial behavior are related to all other problem behaviors.

• Low resistance to peer influences, and having friends who engage in problem behaviors, are common to all problem behaviors.

• All problem behaviors are associated with insufficient bonding to parents, inadequate supervision and communication from parents, and parents who are either too authoritarian or too permissive.

• Living in a poverty area or a high-density urban area is linked with all problem behaviors.

• Rare church attendance is associated with most problem behaviors.

Although no one study has been comprehensive enough to tell the whole story, numerous studies using different sources of data demonstrate that problem behaviors overlap. In general, adolescents engaged in any one are more likely to be engaged in the others. School failure begins at an early age, and once that failure occurs, other events begin to occur. As these high-risk children grow older, substance abuse and sexual activity enter the picture, followed by ever more serious consequences — early childbearing, heavy substance abuse, serious delinquency, and dropping out of school.

A variety of psychosocial factors contribute to problem behavior such as frequent drinking. Adolescents drink for several reasons beyond the desire to become intoxicated: to establish commonality with peers; to demonstrate independence; to express opposition to parents or society; to cope with stress; to achieve a new personal identity; to lubricate social interaction; and to mark the transition to a more mature status. They may use the efforts of alcohol as a kind of self-medication for distress, or to facilitate their social performance, or to "act big" to signify their movement toward adult status.

In careful and systematic studies comparing non-problem drinkers and problem drinkers in adolescence, the problem drinkers place a lower value on academic achievement. They are less religious than their counterparts. They value independence and deviant behavior more than most of their peers do. They value personal independence more than they do academic achievement.

Also, as compared with non-problem drinkers among their peers, they report less compatibility between parents and friends, greater influence of friends on decision making, and greater approval from their friends for problem behavior. More than their counterparts, their drinking is associated with delinquent behavior and marijuana use. They seem to relish being unconventional, perhaps as a reflection of a kind of pseudo-independence. Such characteristics are conducive to a variety of adolescent problems.

One longitudinal study indicates that about half of male adolescent problem drinkers and a quarter of females will become adult problem drinkers. Young adult problem drinkers also manifest a variety of other problems, such as heavy smoking and multiple arrests, as well as higher rates of divorce. The greatest differences in Jessor's longitudinal study are between the abstainers and the drinkers. Apparently, the decision to drink regularly is part of and contributes to a major difference in lifestyle. This is only one line of inquiry that highlights any linkage among adolescent problems. Such linkage deserves a high priority in research, so we can find out how to prevent adolescents from putting themselves at high risk.

Those who smoke and drink in early adolescence are also likely to try unprotected sex and to fail in school. In effect, they are trying out lifestyles that may be exploratory in this phase but all too readily can become entrenched as they move into later adolescence.

What proportion of young adolescents are clearly at risk of slipping into long-term patterns of unhealthy and unproductive lives? Recent estimates indicate that of the 28 million people between the ages of ten and seventeen in the United States, about 7 million are highly vulnerable to the negative consequences of multiple high-risk behaviors such as school failure, substance abuse, and early, unprotected sexual intercourse. So it is reasonable to say that one-quarter of American adolescents fall into a high-risk category. Another 7 million are at moderate risk by virtue of lesser involvement in such behaviors — e.g., occasional rather than regular substance abuse, protected rather than unprotected early sexuality, underachievement in school rather than flunking out.

A task force studying education in early adolescence under the auspices of the Carnegie Council on Adolescent Development assessed the cost of preventable problems. Their findings are sobering.

Dropping Out of School

- Each year's dropouts cost the nation about $260 billion in lost earnings and forgone taxes over their lifetime.

- A male high-school dropout earns $260,000 less than a high-school graduate and contributes $78,000 less in taxes over his lifetime. For a female dropout, the comparable figures are $200,000 and $60,000.

- Unemployment rates for dropouts are more than double those of high-school graduates.

- Each added year of secondary education reduces the probability of public welfare dependency in adulthood by 35%.

Adolescent Pregnancy

- More than $19 billion was spent in 1987 in payments for income maintenance, health care, and nutrition to support families begun by adolescents.

- Babies born to adolescent mothers are at high risk of low birth-weight. Initial hospital care for low-birthweight infants averages $20,000. Total lifetime medical costs for low-birthweight infants average $400,000 per child.

- Of adolescents who give birth, 46% go on welfare within four years; of unmarried adolescents who give birth, 73% go on welfare within four years.

Alcohol and Drug Abuse

- In the eighties, alcohol and drug abuse in the United States cost about $150 billion per year in reduced productivity, treatment, crime, and related costs. If the toll of cigarette smoking is included, the costs are much higher.

Tackling the Problems of Adolescence

The vulnerability of early adolescents to health and educational risks has only recently come into focus. It is essential to move these problems higher on the agenda of scientific research, public education, and institutional innovation. Promising leads exist. We need to identify the programs that are helping to foster responsible innovations. We must find ways to help families and communities foster healthy adolescent development. The present casualties are too high and much of the damage to our adolescents may well prove to be preventable.

There is not the slightest reason to believe that today's young people are less talented or resourceful than their predecessors, but their circumstances are considerably different, and so, too, their tasks and obstacles. To help them learn what they have to learn to survive and flourish and create, we have to understand these circumstances, tasks, and obstacles better than we now do. Then adults can help children and adolescents prepare adequately for adult life and perhaps shape a more humane and compassionate society together.

Works Cited

Bancroft, J., and Reinisch, J.M., Eds. *Adolescence and Puberty*. New York: Oxford University Press, 1990.

Brooks-Gunn, J., and Petersen, A., Eds. *Girls at Puberty: Biological and Psychosocial Perspectives*. New York: Plenum Press, 1983.

Conger, J., and Petersen, A. *Adolescence and Youth: Psychological Development in a Changing World*, 3rd ed. New York: Harper & Row, 1984.

Dash, L. *When Children Want Children: The Urban Crisis of Teenage Childbearing*. New York: William Morrow, 1989.

Dryfoos, J.G. *Adolescents at Risk: Prevalence and Prevention*. New York: Oxford University Press, 1990.

Duany, L., and Pittman, K. *Latino Youths at a Crossroads*. Washington, DC: Children's Defence Fund, 1990.

Erickson, E.H. *Identity: Youth and Crisis*. New York: W. W. Norton, 1968.

Feldman, S.S., and Elliott, G.R. *At the Threshold: The Developing Adolescent*. Cambridge, MA: Harvard University Press, 1990.

Furstenberg, F.F., Jr., Brooks-Gunn, J., and Chase-Lansdale, L. "Teenaged Pregnancy and Childbearing." In *American Psychologist*, vol. 44, no. 2, February 1989.

Hamburg, B.A. "Early Adolescence: A Specific and Stressful Style of the Life Cycle." In *Coping and Adaptation*, G.V. Coelho, D.A. Hamburg, and J.E. Adams, Eds. New York: Basic Books, 1974.

Hamburg, B.A., and Hamburg, D.A. "Stressful Transitions of Adolescence: Endocrine and Psychosocial Aspects." In *Society, Stress, and Disease*, vol. 2, L. Levi, Ed. London: Oxford University Press, 1974.

Hamburg, B.A. "Early Adolescence as a Life Stress." In *Coping and Health*, S. Levine and H. Ursin, Eds. New York: Plenum Press, 1980.

Hayes, C.D., Ed. *Risking the Future: Adolescent Sexuality, Pregnancy, and Childbearing*, vol. I. Washington, DC: National Academy Press, 1987.

Hayes-Bautista, D.E., Schink, W.O., and Chapa, J. *The Burden of Support: Young Latinos in an Aging Society*. Stanford, CA: Stanford University Press, 1988.

Healthy People 2000. U.S. Department of Health and Human Services Public Health Service, Superintendent of Documents, U.S. Government Printing Office, Washington (PHS) 91-50212, 1990.

Hein, K. *Issues in Adolescent Health*: An Overview. Working paper for the Carnegie Council on Adolescent Development, Washington, DC, 1988.

Hendee, W. R., Ed. *The Health of Adolescents*. San Francisco: Jossey-Bass Publishers, 1991.

Hetherington, E.M. "Coping with Family Transitions: Winners, Losers, and Survivors." In *Child Development*, vol. 60, 1-15, 1989.

Highlights of National Adolescents School Health Survey: Drug and Alcohol Use. Rockville, MD: U.S. Department of Health and Human Services, 1988.

Hurrelmann, K., and Losel, F., Eds. *Health Hazards in Adolescence*. New York: Walter de Gruyter, 1990.

Injury in America: A Continuing Public Health Problem. National Research Council, Commission on Life Sciences, Committee on Trauma Research and the Institute of Medicine. Washington, DC: National Academy Press, 1985.

Jessor, R. "Critical Issues in Research on Adolescent Health Promotion." In *Promoting*

Adolescent Health: A Dialogue on Research and Practice, T.J. Coates, A.C. Peterson, and C. Perry, Eds. New York: Academic Press, 1977.

Jessor, R., and Jessor, S.L. *Problem Behavior and Psychosocial Development: A Longitudinal Study of Youth.* New York: Academic Press, 1977.

Johnston, L.D., O'Malley, P.M., and Bachman, J.G. *Drug Use, Drinking, and Smoking: National Survey Results from High School, College, and Young Adult Populations 1975-1988.* Rockville, MD: U.S. Department of Health and Human Services, 1989.

Lancaster, J., and Hamburg, B.A., Eds. *School-Age Pregnancy and Parenthood: Biosocial Dimensions.* Hawthorn, NY: Aldine de Gruyter, 1986.

Lerner, R.M. and Foch, T.T., Eds. *Biological-Psychosocial Interactions in Early Adolescence,* Hillsdale, NJ: Lawrence Erlbaum Associates, 1987.

Millstein, S.G., and Litt, I.F. "Adolescent Health and Health Behaviors." In *At the Threshold,* S.S. Feldman, and G.R. Elliott, Eds. Cambridge, MA: Harvard University press, 1990.

Patterson, G.R., DeBaryshe, B.D. and Ramsey, E. "A Developmental Perspective on Antisocial Behavior." In *American Psychologist,* special issue, vol. 44, no. 2, February 1989.

Petersen, A.C. "Adolescent Development." In *Annual Review of Psychology,* vol. 39, 583-607, 1988.

Pusey, A.E. "Behavioural Changes at Adolescence in Chimpanzees." In *Behaviour,* 115 (3-4), 1990.

Runyan, C.W., and Gerken, E.A. "Epidemiology and Prevention of Adolescent Injury." In *Journal of the American Medical Association,* vol. 262, no. 16, October 27, 1989.

Teenage Pregnancy: An Advocate's Guide to the Numbers. Washington, D.C.: Children's Defense Fund, 1988.

Walters, J.R. "Transition to Adulthood." In *Primate Societies.* B. Smuts, et al., Eds. Chicago: University of Chicago Press, 1986.

Williams, T. *The Cocaine Kids.* Reading, MA: Addison-Wesley, 1989.

World Health Organization. *The Health of Youth.* Technical Discussions, WHO, Geneva, Switzerland, May 1989.

Youth Indicators, 1988: Trends in the Well-Being of American Youth. Washington, DC: U.S. Department of Education, 1988.

Zill, N. "Behavior, Achievement, and Health Problems Among Children in Stepfamilies: Findings from a National Survey of Child Health." In *Impact of Divorce, Single-Parenting, and Stepparenting on Children,* E.M. Hetherington and J. Arasteh, Eds. Hillsdale, NJ: Lawrence Erlbaum Associates, 1988.

CHAPTER 4

CARING WITH ADOLESCENTS IN CRISIS

G. Wade Rowatt

Pastors, parents, professional counselors, youth ministers, teachers, lay volunteers and other helping professionals are encountering adolescents in increasing numbers with more serious crises. Adolescent crises have some similarities to adult crises, but the uniqueness of the adolescent's psychosocial and faith context requires a specific understanding of the adolescent in the Space Age dilemma. Furthermore, an understanding of oneself in relationship to one's own adolescent issues and experiences facilitates caring with adolescents in crisis.

INTRODUCTION

The essay will provide readers with an understanding of adolescent crises while convincing them to participate with adolescents in their crises. In order to participate one must examine oneself and the principles which guide one's ministry. A final purpose of the essay, developing practical approaches to caring for adolescents in crisis, will provide a starting point for the reader's own creativity. The understanding and principles will be more universal; however the practical approaches need to be custom fitted for each context. Readers' creativity, ingenuity and imagination undoubtedly will produce new approaches for caregiving with teens.

The material for this essay grows from a quarter of a century of attempting to work with teenagers. The author has been a high school mathematics teachers, a youth minister in a large suburban southern congregation, a pastor of a small town Midwest church, a chaplain in a hospital, and a pastoral counselor. A more serious inquiry into the nature of adolescence began with a sabbatical leave that produced *Pastoral Care with Adolescents in Crisis*, a textbook for those wanting indepth study in the art of caregiving with teens. For 13 years, the author wrote an "Ann Landers" type column in a teenage magazine, *event*. More recently, a book to parents, *How to Talk with Teenagers*, has provided an opportunity to research more carefully the family dimension of adolescent crises more carefully.

In addition to professional experience and knowledge from behavioral science and ministry, the author's own personal involvement with adolescents informed this material. At various times, the author's family has cared for two adolescent foster child-type situations and has raised twins who have just completed their adolescent years.

Participating in Adolescent Crisis Issues

"Understanding adolescent crisis issues" could well be the heading of this section. However, understanding falls short of the full involvement necessary to understand. Participating in adolescent crisis connotes the necessity of engaging oneself more deeply with adolescents in their world. It is a broader commitment to an "I-Thou" relationship (Martin Buber) with the adolescent world. To understand adolescents requires a commitment to know them and even beyond knowing them, to struggle with them. One must be a participant-observer in the matrix of their relationships. The detachment frequently proposed for professionals involved in crisis counseling does not work as well with adolescents. The theoretical detachment of classical psychoanalysis misses the adolescent psyche.

To understand the adolescent we must first understand the adolescent's context. Adolescence itself is a modern phenomenon. Obviously the teen years following puberty have existed since the beginning of the species. However, adolescence as a life stage begins with the Reformation and the Industrial Revolution. In biblical times young men and women were introduced directly into adulthood. Rituals that marked the rite of passage frequently around the age of 13 placed on their shoulders the full responsibility of adulthood. Young women were given in marriage or to religious service, young men were given to be priests, warriors, shepherds and farmers.

With the Industrial Revolution and even more now in the electronic age, adolescence emerges as a time of preparation for adulthood. The changes brought about in society necessitate more training and skill academically and socially in order to participate fully in society. As David Elkind points out in his creative volume, *All Grown Up and No Place to Go*, youth are ready for the real world long before the real world has a place for them. This need for a time to be prepared is more pronounced in industrialized countries. Third world nations and cultures closer to the rhythms of the earth still introduce their adolescents into the adult world earlier and appear to have fewer adolescent crises, i.e., fewer pregnancies out of wedlock, lower adolescent suicide rates, and lower adolescent chemical dependency rates.

The Industrial Revolution soon took the father out of the home and lessened or completely removed his influence on the adolescent's development. The Space Age has made labor a touchpad, push button, electronic experience, and now the mother has followed the father out of the home. Children and adolescents experience less support from their parents in the family system at the very time society is placing more stress upon them. Understanding the adolescent dilemma of more demands and less support underscores the critical nature of involvement on the part of the church and others who dare to care for this segment of society.

Today's Western adolescents have more free time, less supervision, and consequently are searching for real involvement. This situation adds to their consumerism, romanticism, and sometimes even casual attitude toward life.

One factor further complicating the adolescent dilemma is the image created in the media. Adolescents see from commercials, music videos, and movies an image of other adolescents in idealized, romantic worlds where love and attention invade their psyche like invaders on a video screen. Unfortunately the real world does not substantiate this romanticized image of adolescence. In the real world today's teenagers are more lonely, have fewer true friends, and feel less loved. They despair in the face of the discrepancies of the idealized image of the modern teen and their actual experience as a young person.

In a survey for pastoral care with adolescents in crisis, ten issues surfaced as crisis areas for teenagers. Five questionnaires were sent to 250 ministers, counselors, chaplains and youth workers in all 50 states. Approximately 100 questionnaires were returned.

Levels of Need for Care with Adolescents

The following chart lists in order the intensity of the crisis which adolescents experience as ranked by these professional caregivers (Rowatt 12).

Levels of Adolescents Needs

Ranked as Greatest Need	Area of Need
1	Identity Crisis
2	Friendships and peers
3	Parent conflict
4	Drug and alcohol usage
5	Sex related problems
6	Job and vocation
7	Personal depression
8	Faith questions
9	Suicidal thoughts
10	Physical hospitalization

These may be perceived in a different order by the reader. Perhaps the context in which you minister contains elements that would intensify one area of the above concerns. Nevertheless, I believe if you are not dealing with these ten issues that you are missing either a segment of adolescents in your community or perhaps are even closing your eyes to the needs in your group. These headings seem to be rather self-explanatory. (For specific guidance in dealing with a specific crisis you can turn to *Pastoral Care with Adolescents in Crisis*.)

Early Youth Concerns

While I did not survey formally the concerns of youth, I did interview teenagers from Miami to Honolulu, from Texas to Connecticut, and across the spectrum of sizes of communities, from rural communities to small towns to suburban communities and large inner cities. I conducted conversations with small groups and individual teens. Middle and late adolescents voiced concerns a bit differently from early adolescents.

Early adolescents, the group from puberty to age 14 or 15, expressed a number of anxieties. More than a few were anxious about the transition from junior/middle high to high school. There was a fear of social pressure, older adolescents, and perceived uncaring teachers.

A second concern of the younger teen group was losing their parents and feeling less concern from their parents. Several expressed frustration over decreased time with their parents.

Social concerns emerged in a number of young teenagers. While their was an understandable idealizing of the concerns around ecology and their commitment to "save the earth," there was a surprising number concerned about nuclear war and a fear of Space Age destruction. While some voiced a pride in perceived military power, most were fearful for their own lives and safety.

Safety at school emerged as a concern for lower and middle class teens whose confidence in the public schools seems to be eroding quickly. They imagined being confronted by older teens with weapons, or they feared being physically intimated.

Later Youth Concerns

Middle adolescents (age 15 to 17) and late adolescents (age 18 to adulthood) expressed similar concerns with varied degrees of intensity. This group's major concern seemed to be social relationships including dating and friendships. While many of them assumed that most of their peers were happily dating they expressed frustration themselves. Surveys indicate 80% of teenagers want to be dating while fewer than 20% have a date on a regular basis. Group dating seems to be the norm for middle and late adolescents as it used to be for early adolescents.

A profound sense of isolation and loneliness pervades the psyche of many teens. They feel no one really cares. They overgeneralize the acceptance others experience and catastrophize the rejection they experience. [1]

A further concern of middle and late adolescents focused on their families. For the most part they were wanting freedom from their parents but not from their parent's economic support. Middle and late adolescents want to have their cake and eat it too. They want to make all their own decisions and finance them with their parents' support. Materialism seduces many middle class and upper middle class adolescents and not a few from the lower socioeconomic group. Adolescent crime is on the increase because of the pressure to have things. In the face of the existential anxieties of loneliness and separation from parents, accumulating electronic gadgets and gizmos offer some teens a false sense of identity.

A second older teen concern was dealing with dysfunctional parents. While many had been traumatized by the divorce of their parents, a large number felt equally traumatized by living with what I would call dysfunctional parents. The parents did not have sufficient boundaries between the parent role and the child role in the family.

A further concern of late adolescents was being pushed vocationally. This expressed itself in early and middle adolescents as being pressured to excel too soon. A number of teens who felt they were supposed to be "superkids" expressed the feeling that they had to either be at the top of their class or be ashamed. This appeared more pronounced among Asian-Americans than among Afro-Americans or Euro-Americans. Others felt pushed to excel athletically, dramatically, musically, or in whatever area of concern appeared important to their parents. The late adolescents felt pushed to select a vocation or a profession. A few middle adolescents felt that they were to have their college selected and their life goal set by 15 years of age.

Among poverty stricken adolescents, a sense of hopelessness, frustration, and in some cases rage, prevailed. While living in the land of plenty, they experience hunger and poverty. The hopelessness seemed most pronounced among young black males who are not in church. Interestingly enough, there was a high sense of self-esteem and hope among black, churched adolescent males. Generally speaking, black adolescent females expressed more hope from their poverty context than did white adolescent males or females whose family experienced poverty.

It seems that to understand the contemporary adolescent one must understand the dynamics that contribute to the lessening of support systems for teenagers. Also one needs to understand the social pressures as perceived by professionals and adolescents. Finally one needs to understand the adolescent developmental context. (For further reading in understanding the adolescent developmental cycle, see Daniel O. Aleshire, *Understanding Today's Youth*, Broadman Press: Nashville, TN, 1982.)

Perhaps 30-50% of all adolescents will experience some type of crisis in the teen decade. That is, their parents will divorce, they will be hospitalized or depressed, or lonely, or they will be the victim of some tragedy.

PRINCIPLES OF CARING WITH ADOLESCENTS

Principles of caring with adolescents provide a sense of direction in the complexity of the multifaceted problems that encompass problem teenagers. Pastoral principles underscore the unique role of the minister as she or he cares for adolescents. Certainly more troubled adolescents will need the care of other professionals such as family counselors, social workers, and physicians, nevertheless staying theologically grounded underscores the uniqueness of the minister's role. There are three areas of principles that deserve further reflection and discussion: awareness, assessment, and actions.

Our awareness of the nature of our relationships with teens contributes to a sense of mutual trust. However, our capacity as professionals must move us beyond just trust and friendship to the level of assessing accurately the nature of the crisis. After we assess the crisis and community with some clarity that assessment with the teen, then certain actions on our part and theirs must be undertaken for appropriate response to the crisis.

Awareness Principles

Perhaps the most important awareness to take into a ministry context with a teenager is egalitarian partnership. Ministers need to be aware of the adolescent's concern to be treated as an equal. As caregivers offer first their friendship, they communicate respect for the teenager as a human being. This helps confront the "you're a little person" attitude. One needs to be cautious not to take teenagers and their problems too casually. Belittling and talking down to teens reflects the opposite of this egalitarian partnership attitude. Before teens will trust a minister privately this attitude of partnership will need to be communicated publicly through teaching, preaching, and social situations.

The second attitude to carry into an adolescent crisis situation is commitment. The adolescent needs to feel that the minister will stand by them and be on their side regardless of the relationship's direction. Often troubled juveniles are detached from caring adults and therefore need this sense of commitment even more. A few will never have had a durable relationship with an adult, even a parent, that they could trust. Building this bond will be an even more critical variable in crisis management.

Specific ways of expressing the attitude of "I'll stand by you" involves such things as taking initiative in negotiating contacts and appointments, maintaining an interest in their other activities and discussing future events such as graduation with them. If the minister can participate in some of their events such as showing up for a ballgame or appearing in court with them this further underscores an attitude of commitment.

Openness to new issues through a non-defensive poster is a third attitude necessary for ongoing care with adolescents in crisis. Such openness calls for meeting the teenager in his or her world of language and ideas. It may even call for meeting them outside of the office, in their home, at the pizza parlor or on the parking lot. The context of caring for adolescents in crisis may not be the church office, sanctuary, or counseling room, but will more likely need to be a long walk, a casual conversation pacing around the room, or sharing a soft drink in a fast food place. While flexibility is important to the context of the care, it is perhaps even more important in the relationship. While a teenager may be open and willing to respond to a minister's offer of care at one time, but a few days later the adolescent may need to pull back and remain detached. An attitude of openness to let the teenager's mood set the stage for the depth of the conversation strengthens the capacity to care in the midst of a crisis. Care needs to be taken that this openness does not communicate powerlessness on the part of the caregiver. There is still a time for setting limits, drawing the line, and remaining firm, but precautions must be taken not to be rigid.

An attitude of privacy must be maintained at all times. This fourth attitude is a vital principle in caring for adolescents in crisis. Remember certain information such as physical abuse and sexual abuse cannot be maintained in secrecy but must be reported to the legal authorities. Nevertheless, other information such as a broken dating relationship, being fired from a job, having a brush with legal authorities, needs to be held in the strictest of confidence.

Most ministers will find this attitude difficult in their parish setting because of the sense of responsibility to the family and parents. While each person must determine ethically what he or she will hold secret and what must be shared with family or other professions, an attitude of respecting the boundaries of the adolescent's information must be conveyed. Ministers need to communicate clearly with adolescents information that must be shared. It is better to tell the adolescent ahead of time than to have the adolescent discover late that a confidence has been violated. For example, the minister might say, "I feel compelled to inform your parents that you are having these self-destructive thoughts. We must get you some help. I've got to refer you for professional care." Adolescents will respect professional use of confidence. However, they are understandably slow in forgiving a minister who slips in conversation and shares embarrassing information about a date or an awkward social event with other members of the congregation.

A fifth attitude for caring with adolescents is understanding. Simply put, you must know teenagers and communicate to them that you know not only their general plight but their specific problems. Teenagers are often more concerned that their point of view be understood than they are worried about getting their way. Many adolescents cry for understanding from the adult world. They feel adults have forgotten the pain and perhaps never knew the depth of frustration that they experience.

While communicating caring, understanding ministers need to be cautious not to communicate that the adolescent world was the very same for them. While we have some memories from our own adolescent experience, teenagers are put off by attempts to make one-to-one correlations between our adolescent world and theirs. They don't need us to say "It was exactly that way when I was your age" as much as they want to hear, "Tell me what it's like for you. I remember some of those struggles but I'm sure your situation is different."

A final attitude to carry into our ministry with adolescents in crisis is an attitude of sensitivity to gender issues. Boys and girls, men and women, males and females are different! While the universality of personhood calls for equality between men and women, the differences necessitate a respect for uniqueness. Men's identity formation and women's identity formation in pre-Industrial Revolution society had a clarity of roles even though it seems to have neglected equality and respect. Hard work on the part of social and political activists has brought more respect and equality but there is a danger in losing the individuality of the sexes. Ministers need to understand that perhaps a person of the same sex will be needed to discuss some problems with teenagers in crisis. For example, as soon as possible after learning of sexual abuse or rape, a person of the same sex needs to be available to talk with the victim. In providing role models persons of the same gender need to be available in the group. An attitude of respect for gender differences needs to reflect the equality of Scriptures like Galatians 3:28: "There is neither Jew nor Greek, bond nor free, male nor female, for you are all one in Christ Jesus." While these attitudes create an atmosphere necessary for establishing a bond with adolescents in crisis, the capacity to detach one-self and observe carefully the dynamics is necessary for an accurate assessment. Caregivers need to be simultaneously involved in the process of relating to the adolescent and removed from the process enough to assess the nature of the crisis.

Assessment Principles

As the adolescent shares the nature of the crisis the first assessment principle is to avoid projection. Caregivers who do not know themselves well or perhaps are unaware of their own spiritual struggles and psychosocial issues run the danger of seeing their own issues projected on to the screen of the adolescent's life drama. Such "personal issue" blindness makes assessing the adolescent's situation impossible. While delayed adolescent issues may help some youth ministers relate recreationally with the teen world, delayed adolescent struggles handicap caring adults in attempts to respond during crises. While this would be true of emergency crises such as hospitalization, family problems or legal issues, it is perhaps more true of developmental, emerging crises such as turning sixteen, dealing with a vocational decision or handling the grief over a lost love.

A second assessment principle, using your own relationship as a guide to understanding the teen, requires a high level of self-awareness. As the teenager discusses the nature of their crisis, the caregiver develops feelings toward the teenager. Sensitive assessors know how to use these feelings as a guide to understanding how other persons will respond to this teen. For example, one might begin to be hostile or angry toward the teenager asking for help. As these angry feelings emerge, caregivers can ask what about the teenager prompts the hostility and could that same dynamic be contributing to the nature of the crisis? Manipulative teenagers might be sabotaging their own systems of help at home, school or work. When the manipulation appears to the minister as a reason for hostilities, it can be used as a tool or assessment.

A third assessment principle focuses on understanding the developmental stage and issues of the teenager. In emergency crises, developmental issues for the teenager form a lens through which they see the emergency event. For example, if a teenager's key developmental issue is learning to date, concerns about dating may become a primary lens through which they view decisions around their parents' divorce. One teenager chose to live with the father whom she despised rather than move with the mother she loved. Her key issue was that the father was staying in the community and she had begun dating a boy at her school only two weeks before. Knowing the teenager's developmental issue provides vital information in assessing not only the cause and impact of the crisis but also in assessing the probable resolution of the crisis. Remember teens mature at different rates. Knowledge of what is developmentally normal for a given age must be coupled with the ability to hear each youth's own developmental concerns.

A fourth principle takes into account the tension between social pressure and responsibility. In assessing the crisis the caregiver needs to sort out contextual issues from personal issues. For example, a young man who has been arrested for shoplifting may have a personal problem or may in complex ways be reflecting the injustice of his own economic plight. Social factors are a major force in adolescent behavior. Because a minister may be enmeshed in the same social context, assessing such factors can be quite difficult. If there is a pattern of types of crisis among a given adolescent group that should be a "red flag" indicator to the minister that some larger social issue may be impacting all of them. Of course it could be personal peer pressure accounting for the universality of the crisis. For example, if a disproportionate number of teenagers are dealing with suicidal thoughts within a youth group, it could be that they have formed a suicide pact or there could be social pressures generating a pervasive hopelessness in their society.

A fifth assessment principle involves understanding the faith issues and spiritual formation of the adolescent. Assessing the adolescent's religious history is more than looking at a litany of their religious activities. Knowing faith development and spiritual formation processes enables the minister to assess the pilgrimage of each adolescent. Unresolved faith issues may precipitate a crisis. For example, a teenager may become angry at God because a sibling had an accident and God is blamed for it. In anger at God the teenager may begin acting out irresponsibly. (For further discussion of discussing faith issues with teens see, *How to Talk with Teenagers* by Wade Rowatt.)

Assessing faith issues also involves looking at the stage of moral development. Many youth are doing the right things but for the wrong reasons. For example they may be living within the boundaries of acceptable behavior only out of fear of being caught. These youth have not matured to the point of pursuing the right for the sake of love, of self, God and others. Faith and moral development issues are an important part of assessment because of their impact on the youth's decision making process. Decisions concerning response to a particular crisis are often made out of insufficient faith development and immature moral development. (See James Fowler *The Stages of Faith* for expanded discussion.)

A final assessment principle involves assessing the family environment. Effective caregivers know how to assess the adequacy of a family structure and the health of family relationships. Ministers stand in a unique role for such assessment because often they will have a relationship with the family as well as the youth. In most communities ministers still maintain the right of making home visits and on behalf of the adolescent can visit and make an assessment without infringing upon the rights of the family. Using a family genogram produces unusual insight into patterns of family behavior. (See J. C. Wynn for a discussion of the use of genograms in a religious context.)

As caregivers reflect on these assessment principles, they will uncover areas for further professional development. If, for example, one does not understand spiritual formation in adolescents or family dynamics or even developmental issues, further studies in those areas may be necessitated.

Having looked at principles of awareness and assessment, we now turn our attention to some principles that inform our actions in the conversation with an adolescent in crisis. Certain behaviors on the part of the caregiver strengthen the relationship and increase the probability of successful resolution. One does not need to become a skilled psychotherapist in order to help teens in crisis. However, one needs to know when and how to refer troubled adolescents for depth counseling as needed. (See Howard Clinebell's *Basic Types of Pastoral Counseling* for specific guidelines in referral counseling.) Ministers need to develop a list of trusted referral resources. Who in your community can help teens? How do you get a youth into their program? Know your limits and know how to involve other professionals in working with your adolescents whose crises exceed these limits.

Principles for Caring Actions

Specific principles guide one's action into caring with adolescent's during a crisis. These principles, like the principles of awareness and assessment, may vary with the context. Nevertheless, they provide a framework for reference.

Caregivers need to listen twice as much as they talk when assisting adolescents in crisis. Careful listening avoids interruptions, gives undivided attention and frequently checks out the accuracy of understanding.

The importance of listening to the adolescent's hidden message as well as the story line of the crisis cannot be overstated. Adolescents frequently do not know the issues underneath their story line. The hidden message is beyond their awareness frequently. Don't protect, but do offer insights for their consideration.

One teenager underscored the importance of this listening principle when asked to give three guidelines to adults who are helping teenagers. She said: "Listen, listen, and listen."

A second principle for action involves guiding the decision-making process during the crisis. When the crisis event is fresh and emotions are still raw, providing such guidance not only lowers anxiety but also increases the probability that another crisis will not be precipitated by unwise action. For example, one teenager driving recklessly to an emergency room to visit a parent who had been in an accident had an accident himself and was critically injured. Simple guidance or finding someone to drive the panic-stricken youth to the hospital could have perhaps have prevented further tragedy.

In guiding teenagers' decision-making, one must exercise caution not to be a shallow advice-giver. Guidance at its best draws out the issues and clarifies the alternatives, but leaves the decision-making as a responsibility for the youth. After decisions have been finalized youth may need help in planning their implementation.

A third principle for action, being an advocate for the youth, might involve interfacing with other agencies or authority persons on the youth's behalf. Teenagers receive little respect when they confront legal, academic, or even economic systems. This might mean going to court with them or finding someone who can visit with them in the counselor's office at school or accompanying them to discuss the crisis with their parents. Youth need to feel you are present with them emotionally even when you are not physically present.

Youth feel powerless before the complexity of administrative and social systems. It is not that the systems intend to manipulate youth always, but youth may be inexperienced and unaware of how to utilize the system. A danger exists that being an advocate will open one up to being used by the youth. A high degree of self-awareness and reflection can minimize this danger for the caregiver.

A fourth principle, expressing and receiving honest emotions, permits the adolescent to ventilate negative, noxious feelings. By sharing one's own emotions the caregiver models for the adolescent appropriate ways of emotional release. Providing a safe environment for ventilation reduces the probability of the teenager acting out dangerously at a later time.

A few caregivers err on the side of repressing the adolescent's "ranting and raving." While it is understandable that reducing anxiety and controlling the hysteria around a crisis can be important, one must also remember that adolescents need to express their feelings before thinking carefully through the alternatives. Feelings most likely needing to be ventilated will be anger, guilt, fear, disappointment and grief. As these feelings are shared, biblical materials that parallel such emotions maybe helpful to the youth.

A final principle for action is to hold out realistic hope in the midst of the crisis. As religious caregivers, hope is grounded in our system of faith. Likewise, the adolescent's hope must grow realistically from their system of faith. Working within the adolescent's faith parameters is perhaps the only alternative. Teens cannot navigate life from a borrowed perspective on faith. Until they own a faith perspective they remain rather hopeless.

This principle of hope should not minimize the reality of danger but can focus on possibilities for the future. Frequently adolescents look only to the past and feel hopeless about themselves, their environment, and the future. Those who provide care for adolescents in crisis do well to refocus their attention on the future with an attitude of hope.

PRACTICAL CONSIDERATIONS IN CARING WITH YOUTH IN CRISIS

Ministers are ideal persons to respond to the needs of teens in trouble. While ministers may be overlooked by crisis trauma teams in some cases, they are uniquely equipped to deal with youth in times of crisis. For one thing, ministers are the professionals most likely to be exposed to several generations of the family. A minister will know and understand the parents and perhaps the grandparents and extended family in some cases. This unique viewpoint assists in diagnosing the reasons behind the crisis but also provides a unique vantage point when considering alternatives and follow up.

A second reason ministers are uniquely qualified involves their training in biblical and theological foundations. A time of crisis is a time

of questioning one's foundational assumptions. Physicians, social workers, and secular counselors are ill-equipped by training to assist in
reflecting upon life's basic assumptions. Because of the minister's understanding of theological, ethical and philosophical concepts, she or he can
play a unique role in turning the crisis from just another tragic event into
an opportunity for growth not only for the individual youth but also for
the family system.

In the third place, crises often bring broken relationships. And ministers are agents of reconciliation. Due to the minister's awareness of the
dynamics of love, sin, repentance, forgiveness, and reconciliation he or
she can respond at deeper levels when relationships are broken. As agents
for justice and love, ministers model peacemaking and urge families to do
the same.

A final reason for minister's central role in crisis caregiving is their
context for involvement. The church, as an ongoing community of faith,
provides not only a spiritual but also emotional and sometimes physical
sanctuary during the time of the crisis. Existing youth programs can be an
oasis of security for an adolescent recovering from a major crisis.
Outreach programs are frequently used in preventive crisis education
(such as a place to teach sex education, alcohol and drug education, and
dating information). They can also be used for crisis intervention. For
example, a youth group may be utilized to visit a hospitalized teenager.

Groups That Care

Ministers can guide their congregation to provide ongoing groups
that make a difference to teens in crisis. These groups may be informa-
tional, relational or therapeutic. While no church would be expected to
provide all of these services, any church can expand its programs with
appropriate resources.

Churches responding in the survey have indicated success in offering adolescent growth groups where eight or ten adolescents meet and
discuss relevant issues as they bring them up. These groups function on a
non-specific agenda that might include such topics as understanding
today's music, what makes parents act like they do, how to get a date,
how to stop smoking, or is Jesus like the Easter Bunny and Santa Claus.

"Parents of teenagers" support groups have been successful in a
number of churches. These groups usually meet for an hour on Sunday
with a variety of activities. Some discuss books, other share personal incidents, a few have gone through self-guided parenting courses such as
Systematic Training for Effecting Parenting or *Parenting by Grace.*

Churches can provide space for existing groups. Numerous churches offer a place for Alcoholics Anonymous, for Alateen or for Narcotics Anonymous meetings within their facilities. Other self-help groups might include Survivors of Suicide, Compassionate Friends, or a specialized group coping with any type of illness or accident.

Practical Reflections

A number of pragmatic issues were sent to this author by ministers who care for adolescents. Perhaps the most frequently mentioned issue is the necessity to have adequate referral resources available before the crisis. One minister built a referral file when she moved into a new community. She would visit and call the agencies in her community until she had confidence that she knew where to refer persons for a variety of crisis. She had cases for referral that involved finding jobs, receiving medical attention, receiving counseling, and educational guidance. She had even made contact with the local juvenile justice system.

"Include the family as a part of the caregiving" was a recurrent suggestion from pastors. While full time youth ministers more likely focused on the adolescent, pastors saw the need to work with the family as well as the teen. A crisis with an adolescent obviously reverberates throughout the home. While a few pastors seem to neglect the teen and to focus only on the family, most strive for some balance between caring for the family and caring for the young person.

Bad thinking leads to dangerous action. Thinking errors and errors of judgment not only precipitate crises but worsen crises when they go unconfronted. Ministers who care for teenagers will need to help them not "make a mountain out of a molehill" or only see the dark side of the storm clouds. Furthermore, one does well to expose adolescents to the reality that they are not the only persons in crisis. Perhaps it will be necessary to confront their egocentric negative questioning. Some teens will ask, "Why does everything happen to me?" In reality, it doesn't. Care must be exercised not to build a wall between oneself and the teenager as one confronts these errors in thinking. [2]

The Ministerial Black Bag

When physicians made home visits they carried their medical instruments and a limited supply of medication in a black bag. That black bag served as their unique professional identity. Physicians in electronic, modern medical facilities no longer carry a black bag. Similarly, many ministers have lost their professional black bag by trusting exclusively their training in behavioral science when responding to a crisis. Ministers do well to remember the unique power of scripture, prayer and community of faith in responding to adolescents in crisis.

Scriptures can be used most effectively with adolescents in crisis when the adolescents are well informed concerning the scripture. Reminding such a teen of scriptural support can strengthen their faith, hope and love in the time of crisis. However, scriptural stories can be read or perhaps retold in a modern setting in ways that provide strength and support for teens unaware of the Bible. Storytelling can convey scriptural truths, hold the teen's interest, and provide a rapport between the caregiver and the youth. Perhaps when the crisis is most intense the scripture will do little more than inform the approach of the minister and set a context for ministerial identity. However, especially in times of reflecting upon the alternatives available before the team and in times of reflecting upon what was learned from crisis, scriptures play an important role.

Prayer with teens in crisis requires sensitivity. While ritualistic prayer will mean something to youth whose past has been enriched by such experience, youth who are unaccustomed to ritualistic prayers may be turned off, embarrassed or confused or even frightened. In praying with teens in crisis, one does well to ask permission of the teen, reflect the teen's concerns and anxieties in the prayer, and lift up appropriate areas for hope. If a teen feels uncomfortable and requests that the minister not pray, the minister can at least assure the teen that he or she will pray for them in their private time of meditation. Sometimes during this assurance, one can even be specific about the focus of the prayer. For example, one could say something like, "I want you to know I will be praying for you to be able to get a good nights rest, for you to find strength in yourself to face this difficult situation, and for doors to open for getting out of this situation."

The church as a community of faith is perhaps the most undertapped resource for facing crisis. We know that when burdens are shared they diminish in intensity. A caring congregation provides a rich resource for dispersing the pain during a crisis. Persons can still exercise the ministry of presence by simply being with crisis victims. The church can provide individuals to stay with the family, to visit regularly, or perhaps even to open up their own homes for a period of time to members healing from the crisis.

CONCLUSION

This essay has attempted to guide the reader's reflection on participating in crisis issues with teens as it underscored principles of caring with adolescents and offered practical approaches to such care. The issues facing teens in crisis are indeed complex. But we need not despair or abdicate our responsibility of caring only to non-ministerial resources. Ministers are an important part of the crisis team in caring for youth, their families and their friends in times of trouble.

End Notes

[1] For further information concerning cognitive distortions in adolescents, see David Burns, *Feeling Good: The New Mood Therapy.*

[2] Again, see David Burns, *Feeling Good: The New Mood Therapy* for a full discussion of cognitive distortions and approaches to confronting these distortions.

Works Cited

Aleshire, Daniel O. *Understanding Today's Youth.* Nashville: Broadman Press, 1982.

Clinebell, Howard M., Jr. *Basic Types of Pastoral Care and Counseling: Resource for the Minister of Healing and Growth.* Rev. & enl. ed. Nashville: Abingdon Press, 1984.

Elkind, David. *All Grown Up and No Place to Go: Teenagers in Crisis.* Reading, MA: Addison-Wesley Publishing Co., 1984.

Fowler, James W. *The Stages of Faith: The Psychology of Human Development and the Quest for Meaning.* New York: Harper & Row, 1981.

Hiltner, Seward. *Preface to Pastoral Theology.* Nashville: Abington Press, 1958.

Ross, Richard and G. Wade Rowatt, Jr. *Ministry with Youth and Their Parents.* Nashville: Convention Press, 1986.

Rowatt, G. Wade, Jr. *Pastoral Care with Adolescents in Crisis.* Louisville: Westminster/John Knox Press, 1989.

Wynn, J. C. *Family Therapy in Pastoral Ministry.* San Francisco: Harper & Row, 1982.

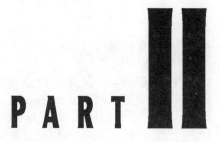

PART II

THE MINISTER AND PASTORAL CARE

Overview

Ministers must be sensitive enough to feel with people, yet strong enough to withstand pressure. When ministers are in tune with themselves, they can touch people in beautiful ways, but when they are out of tune with themselves, not even the Lord can make music with them... No one expects a minister to be perfectly sensitive, strong, and in tune, but everyone expects a minister to function at least adequately, if not well, in most situations (Cavanaugh).

In the next section of the *Guides to Youth Ministry: Pastoral Care*, we examine the need for pastoral care of youth ministers and all those who respond to the call to minister in today's church. We will address key elements for fine tuning the strength and sensitivity of those who advocate for youth, as well as identify skills for competent helping.

In Chapter 5, David Switzer answers two basic questions: "How is it that our response to God is also understood as a commitment to serving persons? How do we see ourselves as Christian helpers and why?" Switzer reflects on the biblical basis for caring and then defines the caring process as "essential for truly human life in the world." He finally identifies self-evaluation, patience, trust, honesty, humility, hope, and courage as significant elements of human caring and how these ingredients need to be woven into our ministry.

Michael Cavanaugh continues this reflection in Chapter 6 with an in-depth look at the psychologically healthy minister and the pastorally effective minister. He believes self-knowledge, self-esteem, self-actualization, and self-fulfillment are critical to ministerial health. Cavanaugh also believes that ministers must work to become more pastoral through a healthy spirituality, motivation, honesty, sensitivity, presence, intellectual competence and approachability. His thoughts are worth a careful reading by all.

This section concludes with Thomas Hart's thoughts on the helper as sacrament and the need to infuse all we do with the principle of sacramentality. He then focuses on the role of the helper in four ways: listening, loving, companioning, and being oneself. Hart concludes with what a helper "is not" — keeping us realistic and balanced!

CHAPTER 5

WHAT DOES IT MEAN TO SAY THAT WE CARE?

David K. Switzer

Regardless of the precise way in which we conceptualize and talk about our motivation for entering and continuing in our ministry in the Church, how much emphasis we place on God's initiative and our response to God's call, whether we phrase the central direction of what we are doing in terms of serving God, almost all of us are also quite aware of our sincere desire to be helpful to persons.

There are two sets of questions to raise in response to this declaration, however. The first of these is, "How is it that our response to God is also understood as a commitment to serving persons? How do we see ourselves as Christian helpers, and why? Why *do* we care?"

There is a second set of questions that we must answer as honestly as we can. "We *want* to be helpful, but *are* we really? To what extent? How much? To what percentage of people with whom we come in contact? To the extent that we *are*, what are the ingredients of our helpfulness? In instances when we are not helpful, why not? What is it that we need in order to be most helpful to the greatest number of people the largest percentage of the time?"

This chapter will attempt to address the issue of how it is that our response to God is also understood as a commitment to serving persons. Why do Christians care? What does it mean to say that we care?

THE BIBLICAL BASIS FOR CARING

My first response to the question of why we care is quite commonplace, even self-evident.

It all begins with the total history of the coming into being of the Jewish people and their covenant with God, God's initiative in promising to make of them a great nation and their promise to be God's people, to be obedient to God. This covenant was reflected in their cohesiveness as a people, their group commitment, their sense of relation to one another. This in turn was demonstrated in their worship of God, the dramatic acts celebrating both their covenant with God and their relationship with one another. The covenant was also the source of their moral laws, principles governing their behavior toward one another. Gradually, God's reality broke into their awareness that God was one and that the one God was the Lord of all people, not just of the Jews themselves. However, as we all know, the Old Testament is not just an account of their loyalty to God, but it also contains the many descriptions of occasions of their breaking the covenant by their disobedience.

At a time when, as a result of their being conquered by another nation and their own nation's ceasing to exist as a viable political unit in 586 B.C., one prophet, whose writings we find in Isaiah 40-66, presented the picture of a small group of Jews who would remain loyal to God in the midst of their defeat, their exile, their trials, their suffering. Those who remained faithful to their covenant with God even at this time were conceived of as being God's suffering servant in restoring the relationship between God and the rest of the people. It was their faithfulness that God would use in bringing them into being once again as a whole people. This vivid and moving description of the Suffering Servant was not the only way in which the Jewish people came to conceive of God's future dramatic acts in history to restore them as a people through a specially chosen agent, God's Messiah, nor was it necessarily the predominant one, but it was there as a part of their tradition, their faith.

Into this people and this faith Jesus was born. The New Testament writers make it clear that Jesus was remembered as one who sought and did the will of God. His obedience led him to the proclamation of the coming kingdom of God, what many scholars think to be the unifying theme of Jesus' whole life. His obedience to God and his looking to the coming kingdom led him to a series of very concrete acts which ministered to the physical, emotional, and spiritual needs of persons while he was also developing around him a community of faith.

The early Christian Church, those of Jesus' own generation and the generation to follow, were also a community of faith, faith in the same God that the Jews had known as Yahweh. Now, however, they were unable to conceive of God and God's activity, God's will and purpose, apart from the life and ministry of Jesus. If we think of the word Christ, the anointed one, as meaning the person who performs the acts of God in the midst of human events, and Jesus as being the one who performs this function of God in human history in a definitive, decisive, and irreplaceable way, then the word "incarnation" takes on a clearer meaning. It is operationally defined.

Jesus, in obedience to the will of God, was the ministering servant of God, the physical body, the activity of Christ. After Jesus' death, the disciples were brought back into community by their experience of the continued life of Christ in their midst, that is, their memory of Jesus and the immediate presence of the Holy Spirit as one inseparable experience. They came to be known as the Church, and they understood their existence in the world as directed toward performing the same function as Jesus himself. That is, in a literal sense, they, the Church, also became the physical Body of Christ. Their purpose in being as a community was to seek and do the will of God, in their quality of life with one another in the world revealing the loving, suffering, redeeming God to the world. They proclaimed and began to act out the life of the coming kingdom of God. This function had clearly been shown in the ministry of Jesus as he had revealed God, indeed, had brought or conveyed God to persons by his accepting the role of Suffering Servant, meeting the needs of the total person, existing on behalf of persons.

Without a doubt, the early Church saw the healing of human ills as being a primary emphasis within their total reason for being since they depicted Jesus' servanthood so frequently in these terms. While the healing of persons was portrayed very clearly in all the gospels it is done very dramatically in Mark, where in the first ten chapters only chapter four has no reference to healing. In the other nine there are a variety of pictures:

several detailed descriptions of particular persons being healed, or general statements such as, "And he healed many persons." Sometimes it would be the other person's initiative to which Jesus responded. On other occasions it would be his initiative in turning aside from other activities to meet an immediate need which he perceived. He used different words and actions. Different types of disorders were healed. The personal ministry to individuals in a variety of kinds of distress, not only healing but also responding to those in grief, forgiving those who seemed to be caught in a trap of self-depreciating and self-negating behavior, all of these healing actions clearly must have been understood by the early Church as being in harmony with and supportive of the proclamation of the kingdom of God and a part of the caring for one another that was to be characteristic of the life of the kingdom.

The words of Isaiah, which were used as Jesus' initiatory declaration at the beginning of his public ministry as reported in Luke 4:16-21, seem then to be central to the *Church's* self-understanding and its acting out of their faith:

> The Spirit of the Lord is upon me, because he has anointed me to preach good news to the poor. He has sent me to proclaim release to the captives and recovering of sight to the blind, to set at liberty those who are oppressed, to proclaim the acceptable year of the Lord.

This is the way in which Jesus understood his mission in obedience to God. This is God's purpose for the church. This mission is literally who we are. It is our reason for being.

In coming into being as Church, the Church is inherently concerned for persons, for the alleviation of their sufferings, for their health and wholeness. We today as the Church of Jesus Christ are called upon to perform our ministry in these areas with the same dedication and vigor and we are called upon to do it with competence. What we refer to as pastoral care in the Church, our concrete acts of caring for one another, is one important way of acting out the ministry of Jesus in obedience to God and the world today, a way of giving our lives for one another, of being servants. This is why we care. The Church is by definition, as a result of God's initiative in caring for us, the caring community.

A Definition of Caring

To this point we have discussed our motivation and our purpose in caring as they are drawn from our faith. But what does it mean to care? In some of the groups I often participate, the word care is used frequently.

For example, I ask students at the beginning of many courses to list their three major strengths which they see as contributing to what they say they want to do as ministers. Almost all of them say as a way of communicating one of their strengths, "I'm a caring person," or "I genuinely care about people." More and more it seems to be a "pop" word, an "in" word. Unfortunately though, the caring to which they are referring has usually been difficult for many of these people to define or describe in any clear-cut concrete way when asked to do so. It seems as if it's just a sense that we have of ourselves or a feeling of ours, something that we can just exude, with the faith that is supposed to carry some magical powers in helping people.

What is caring, anyway? It's obviously not just a Christian word. One person who has sought to elaborate a definition of human caring and its meaning for human life from a purely secular point of view is Milton Mayeroff. By secular, I mean that he makes no reference to any religious experience or religious writings whatsoever. What he does do is to analyze basic human experience itself. The result of that analysis seems to be entirely applicable to *pastoral care*, as well as to other forms of caring within and by the community of faith, how we conduct ourselves in all our relationships with one another, in our preaching, educational practices, business and program planning meetings, what activities we choose to carry out in the Church and community and how we go about executing these.

Mayeroff states:

> To care for another person, in the most significant sense, is to help (that person) grow and actualize himself.... (It) is the antithesis of simply using the other person to satisfy one's own needs. The meaning of caring...is not to be confused with such meanings as wishing (another person) well, liking...or simply having an interest in what happens to another. Also, it is not an isolated feeling or a momentary relationship, nor is it simply a matter of wanting to care for some person. Caring, as helping another grow and actualize himself, is a process, a way of relating to someone that involves development (1).

As he elaborates this definition in more detail, Mayeroff emphasizes that caring is both a persistent *attitude* toward persons and concrete *acts*. Caring and being cared for is essential for truly *human* life in the world, and our own caring for others has the impact of helping us find our place in the world's scheme of things. Mayeroff calls it being "in place in the world" (2). Caring is both an organizing and unifying force in the life of the person who is caring, thus a contribution to the growth and actualization of the one who cares as well as to that of the one being cared for.

In order to care for another in these terms, he says, we experience the other

as an extension of myself and at the same time as something [Shouldn't he have said *someone*?] separate from me that I respect in his own right.... Instead of trying to dominate and possess the other, I want him to grow in his own right, or...to be himself, and I feel the other's growth as bound up with my own sense of well-being (3-4).

Mayeroff states the fundamental principle of caring quite clearly, and this is something which I believe that we need to take *very* seriously and use as a test of our own words and behaviors as Christians as we respond to the needs of others.

In helping the other to grow I do not impose my own direction; rather, I allow the direction of the other's growth to guide what I do, to help determine how I am to respond and what is relevant to such response. I appreciate the other as independent in his own right with needs that are to be respected (5).

There are several things to note about such a statement which I hold to be absolutely essential for caring, and which, as a Christian reading the documents of the early Church, I understand to be Jesus' attitude and behavior toward people. To respect the other persons' unique needs, that particular individual's potential, and to allow and encourage the other person's freedom in decision making does not imply that we are valueless ourselves, or that we should pretend to be, or that we must never share our values and convictions and experiences and faith with one another. In fact, it's absolutely essential that we never lose touch with who it is that we genuinely are as Christian persons as we engage with another in caring for that person. But as a result of valuing *our* values, being aware of needing to have *our* needs met, cherishing and exercising *our* freedom, true caring *must* mean encouraging the growth of just such experiences in the other.

Preaching and worship, Christian education, evangelism, other programming in the Church, our involvement with others in pastoral situations, regardless of the differing forms and specific purposes, are all essentially witnessing, the sharing of experience in an attitude and with acts of love. It is a contradiction in intent and goals if we are coercive and manipulative. Therefore, to seek to impose our own goals, purposes, values, programs, faith, to manipulate or to coerce, however subtly and smoothly, is a failure to trust the basic process of human development within relationships, and, more importantly, the failure to trust the power of the Holy Spirit in human life. We cannot trick people or lead people by the nose into personal growth and change, into significant decisions in their lives, into growth in Christian faith, or into the kingdom itself. The *attempt* to do so is *not* Christian or even human caring.

After all, the process of caring itself as an attitude and relationship as well as concrete facilitating words and acts inevitably produces the greatest potential for the growth of the other person's capacity to care: to care properly for oneself and for persons and causes beyond oneself. No one ever grows without becoming freer, more self-determining, choosing his or her own values and ideals and commitments grounded in his or her own actual experience.

But it is important for us to be aware constantly that *we*, as those who are caring for the other, are a significant *part* of *that* person's experience, and our total set of experiences are a vital part of who we are. Therefore, sharing ourselves in an open and honest way with the other is an essential part of the process of caring. The effectiveness of such sharing is, of course, dependent upon sensitive timing and upon a form which does not seek to impose upon the other.

THE INGREDIENTS OF CARING

Mayeroff lists several major ingredients of caring which flesh out the definition which he has so well begun (9-20). In presenting these elements of caring I have made a change in the heading of one of his categories and the particular ordering of them, have summarized his points, making some modifications in his wording, and have added brief explanations at some points.

1. *Knowledge*: an understanding of the other person's needs and the competence to respond constructively to them. Good intentions and loving feelings do not guarantee either understanding or competence.

2. *The Capacity for Self-Evaluation*: the ability to look critically at our own behavior in relationship to the other person. Have we helped? If so, what was helpful? If not, what was missing in our response? This type of self-evaluation is absolutely necessary for our ability to maintain or to modify our behavior in order to be of the greatest help to the other.

3. *Patience*: staying with the person as she or he is enabled to grow at her or his own time and pace. This patience refers not only to time but also to space, whatever combination is necessary of being physically with the other, speaking or listening, sitting with the other and sharing in the silence, or of actually physically withdrawing in order to allow for the other person's process of assimilation of thoughts and feelings.

4. *Trust*: trust in the process, the relationship, the other person's possibilities (and for us as Christians though Mayeroff makes no reference to it at all trust in the power of the Holy Spirit). Trust also involves not *over*-doing for another, not *over*-protecting the other.

5. *Honest*: seeing oneself and the other as we actually are and not as we would *like* to present ourselves or the other as we would *like* that person to be. In the moment of helping, it is critical for us to be able to see both ourselves and the other only as we actually are, neither more nor less.

6. *Humility*: never allowing ourselves to think that we know all there is to know about the other person or ourselves or how to help in this particular instance, the recognition of our own limitations and our need to be alert and open to learning more about ourselves and the other.

7. *Hope*: in regard to what will happen to and for the other person as a result of our caring.

> hope is not an expression of the insufficiency of the present in comparison with the sufficiency of a hoped for future; it is rather an expression of the plenitude of the present, a present alive with a sense of the possible...it is hope for the realization of the other *through* my caring (19).

8. *Courage*: a necessary prerequisite for the hope just described. There is a risk involved in investing ourselves as we do in caring for another without knowing the outcome. We always lay down some part of our lives for the other in the helping process. Courage is going into the unknown with another. We don't know what will happen to the other person, what he or she will decide to do, what he or she will become, not even what changes will occur to us ourselves.

These are some of the significant elements of human caring. They can be identified from a close and sensitive observation of our own experience and the experience of others. They can be noted and described completely without explicit reference to the Christian faith, although in the context of presenting Mayeroff's definition, I have made several such references. However, when we look at this concept of caring and we place it in the context of the brief review of the biblical material made earlier, we see that caring is *pastoral* when it is not merely one person's caring for another, as Mayeroff has described, but when such caring is *an expression of the whole life and purpose of the Christian community.* Just as Jesus' caring was intertwined with his proclamation of the kingdom of God and was a foretaste of the life of the kingdom, so is the caring of the community of faith today. *Pastoral* caring is defined by the whole event of Jesus' life, death, and resurrection, culminating in the coming into being of the church, with its mission understood in the words of Isaiah as recorded in Luke 4:18-19. Thus, a pastor is any person who is specifically designated by any means as being representative of the Church. The person who is ordained is obviously set aside in a special way by the community of faith so that the person's vocation is to serve and represent the Church on a full-time basis and to be the usual administrator of its sacraments. But, as has been pointed out earlier, non-ordained professional church workers (deacons, diaconal ministers, certified directors of Christian education, music, etc.) also serve and represent the community of faith. In addition, other lay persons may, for longer or shorter periods of time, be asked to represent the Church in particular types of services. The word "pastoral" is appropriate to them also when they are performing these designated functions.

Caring: Agape and Empathy

In order to complete (for the purposes of this chapter) a definition of *why* we care and what it means to care, I'd like to try to link the etymological origin of our present word *care* with *agape*, love, as we find it used in the New Testament, and also with *empathy.* According to the *Oxford Dictionary*, the word "care" comes from the Old Gothic word *kara.* As a noun it meant something like mental suffering, grief, a burdened state of mind, or a matter or object of concern. In its verb form, it meant to sorrow or grieve, to be troubled about. That seems to convey that caring is somehow to suffer or grieve with someone, to carry a burden for or along with the person, to be troubled alongside another.

The noun and verb forms of *agape* in its non-New Testament usage conveyed the meaning of love, kindness, generous or spontaneous goodness. Its New Testament usage came to mean primarily, though not exclusively, benevolence to one's neighbors which was manifested in concrete actions. (Some scholars tell us that the word *philia* seems in a number of places in the New Testament to contain within it the meaning of *agape* [Furnish 1972, 134, 231.]) *Agape*-love means something like "action for the well-being of another, regardless of feeling or the nature of the relationship." In acting for the well-being of your neighbor or your enemy, you may not necessarily become friends or feel affection.

We see, therefore, that caring and *agape* love were not identical in their original root meanings, but for the Christian they are clearly linked, both scripturally and dynamically. John 21:15-17 portrays Jesus as asking Simon Peter three times, "Do you love me?" Peter responds each time, "Of course, You know that I love you." (In this interchange, both of the Greek words for love are used at different points.) Each time Jesus directs, "Then feed, or take care of, my sheep." The total message seems to be, "If you truly know my love for you, then you will love me, and *then* you will obey my commandments. You will love one another; you will feed my sheep." You will become literally a pastor, the word pastor meaning originally to feed and later expanded to mean to take care of a flock. *Agape* and caring for God's people are inseparably connected in the New Testament.

Dynamically that which links caring and *agape* seems to be empathy. What does it mean to care? To care means that to some extent we see ourselves in another person. There is *no one* with whom we don't have some point of identification. It's not just, "there but for the grace of God go I," but much closer to the truth, "There go I!" This point of contact with another human being allows us the possibility of viewing the world, events, life from the perspective *of* that person. Without the capacity to understand another person and that person's world as if we were in some sense that person, without entering into the life and world of another, we cannot truly care and most effectively act for that person's well-being. I certainly don't mean to imply that in entering into another's world and trying to view what goes on from that person's point of view we lose our own identify and perspective, nor do I mean that we somehow should be able to have the same reactions as the other person as we are taking her or his perspective. It does mean increased knowledge, understanding, genuine compassion, patience, trust, humility, hope, courage, as some of these were defined earlier. To be empathetic, to understand another person in this way, also offers some concrete guidelines as to how to respond most helpfully and competently with words to the other person and with other actions on behalf of the other. Caring as "suffering with" becomes *agape*: effective, concrete acts that assist the growth and actualization of the other.

Care, empathy, and *agape* love are like one another in two other ways. First, I've already pointed out that one of the goals of caring is that the other person experience an increase in his or her own ability to care. Empathy, too, as a characteristic of many human beings, is itself both a primary means and a major goal of particular forms of a helping process. Likewise, *agape*, an attitude toward others which expresses itself in concrete acts on their behalf, is a power which has the tendency to produce a like response in the other. "We love, because God first loved us" (1 Jn 4:19).

Second, it isn't sufficient merely to *feel* caring or to *want* to care, to *be* empathetic, to *have* loving feelings or *wish* that we did. All of these require, in order to complete their definitions and to be effective in assisting the growth of another, their open expression in words and often in other acts, words and acts appropriate to the condition and situation of this particular person or group of persons at this particular time. The need of the helping person is not merely a certain attitude and certain feelings, but *competence in the behaviors of helping.*

So, pastoral care is the type of caring which we've defined as an expression of the life of the Christian community, or of a person or persons who are representative of the community, when it is acting out God's purpose in the life, death, and resurrection of Jesus in and for the world. Pastoral caring is one clear expression of *agape* love, the attitude toward others on our part which is representative of the "being-for-others" of God as God is known in Jesus Christ.

There is one final thing that this response to God's grace as we know it in Christ compels me to say at this point. Pastoral responses to people in situations of intense human need, pastoral emergencies, are essential to the internal life of the Church and to the Church's witness to the world, our servanthood in the name of the suffering servant, but I definitely *do not* want to be misunderstood as affirming that pastoral care in emergency and other situations is the only, or even, in many instances, the most important or appropriate form of the Church's servanthood. Not at all! Pastoral care is not the only way in which healing is brought about. There are many sources of separation, many forms of alienation, many varieties of brokenness within the human family: between the Church and the world, between nations and between races, between individual persons and within persons. There are many different forms and causes of suffering. There are literally multitudes of people in the world whose suffering and personal and social deprivation arise from the personal, social, political, and economic restrictions which are forced upon them by the structures of society, by the greed and fear of some of those in positions of wealth and power and privilege who wish to maintain their positions at any cost. There are large numbers of people who are pushed into an existence on the fringe of the mainstream of their society by those either in the majority or who as a minority control the power. Therefore *agape* love, caring as Christians, not only leads us to visit the sick and dying, minister to the bereaved, support the emotionally disturbed, help the alcoholic and abusers of other drugs, counsel persons and couples and families in distress but also thrusts us into the midst of a variety of actions necessary to reduce the prejudice and discrimination and tendencies toward oppression *within* us and *around* us, even in the organization of our whole society and even of our church itself.

SUMMARY

This chapter has sought to clarify and to elaborate in detail the source of the Church's motivation for trying to respond helpfully to persons and families and other groups in their extremities of life as well as on occasions of less pressing need. Those of us who are in places of designated leadership in the Church may rather naturally as human beings seek out or respond to those persons in such situations. In addition, however, as Christians we are also:

1. Being obedient in feeding Christ's lambs, being servants as Jesus was a servant, as God called him and calls us to be. Thus we're literally participating in the life of Christ himself as we suffer with those who suffer, weep with those who weep, rejoice with those who rejoice, sharing our time and energies and sensitivity and skills and faith;

2. Making most possible an openness of the other person or persons to growth in faith, growing in faith ourselves in the process;

3. Contributing to the edifying, the building up the body of Christ, equipping it for fuller and more effective service and witness to Christ in the world.

Works Cited

Mayeroff, Milton. On Caring. New York: Harper & Row, 1971.

Furnish, Victor Paul. *The Love Command in the New Testament*. Nashville: Abingdon Press, 1972.

CHAPTER 6

THE PSYCHOLOGICALLY AND PASTORALLY EFFECTIVE MINISTER

Michael E. Cavanaugh

A violin is a musical instrument that is both sensitive and strong. It is sensitive in that it is affected by the slightest touch, and it is strong because its strings can withstand a good deal of pressure. A violin must be continually and properly tuned to be played well, for if it is not, even the finest violinist cannot call forth beautiful music from it.

As an instrument of the Lord, a minister shares these qualities with a violin. Ministers must be sensitive enough to feel with people yet strong enough to withstand pressure. When ministers are in tune with themselves, they can touch people in beautiful ways, but when they are out of tune with themselves, not even the Lord can make music with them.

There is one area in which the above analogy does not hold. While someone must continually tune the violin, the minister alone is responsible for keeping himself or herself in tune.

No one expects a minister to be perfectly sensitive, strong, and in tune, but everyone expects a minister to function at least adequately, if not well, in most situations. To do this requires more than good intentions and hard work. *As One Who Serves* states the matter clearly and succinctly.

> A person who is a servant leader is expected to be a healthy, maturing person.... In reality, the dimensions or responsibilities of [the minister] as a servant leader are realizable only in the context of the [minister] as a person. Such development includes the emotional, intellectual, and spiritual dimensions of growth (1).

It is toward this end that the present chapter is written. The first part of the chapter deals with some of the aspects of being a psychologically healthy minister; the second part discusses some of the qualities of a pastorally effective minister. The concepts in this chapter are targets to shoot for, goals on which to focus. No minister fully possesses all the qualities that will be discussed, but all ministers should possess them to a greater, rather than a lesser, degree if they realistically expect to be effective instruments of the Lord.

Aspects of a Healthy Sense of Self

The "self" has rarely enjoyed a positive place in Christianity. In its appropriate concern with the sins of selfishness and self-indulgence, the Church overshot the mark and enjoined Christians to become "selfless." Thus the self has often been viewed as a significant obstacle to charity, spirituality, and eternal happiness. Selfless people denied and abrogated their selves to "higher" pursuits. In fact, during one period in Church history, people — many of whom were later to be canonized — publicly vied with each other to see who could best humble his or her self.

Although the concerns of the Church were valid, they tended to cause the Church to throw out the baby with the bath. We now realize that a selfless person is no more apt to be a good Christian than is a selfish one. As with most human behaviors, virtue lies in moderation.

From a personal standpoint, to ignore or disparage the self is to treat poorly a beautiful gift from God. It is far more appropriate to nourish, protect, and celebrate the self than it is to torture it or allow it to die through neglect. From an interpersonal point of view, ignoring the self is analogous to an ambulance driver ignoring and mistreating the engine of his ambulance, even though he does so because he is busy transporting people to the hospital. Sooner or later, the ambulance is likely to run out of gas or fail mechanically and threaten the safety of the very people the driver is trying to help. No one would view an ambulance driver who takes good care of his ambulance as selfish; nor would it be proper to view a minister who takes good psychological care of his or her self as selfish.

Like all Christians and all human beings, ministers have not only the right but the responsibility to celebrate their selves and to take proper care of them, both for their own welfare and the welfare of others. It is virtually impossible for a minister who attends properly to his or her self to experience burnout or other psychological problems. This type of thinking is not new, nor do its roots lie in humanism, personalism, modernism, or psychogism. One need only look to Jesus and the healthier of the saints to see that there is good precedent for proper attention to the self.

Self-Knowledge In Four Dimensions

"Know thyself," said Socrates. The possession of self-knowledge is the first aspect of a healthy sense of self. The self is analogous to a terrain that is smooth in parts, rough in others, and also marbled with gullies and dead-end roads. A minister who has an accurate self-map will arrive at his or her destination with a minimum amount of difficulty. If clouds of defense mechanisms cover parts of the terrain, a minister will experience inordinate difficulties, and may fall, get lost, or arrive at a dead end.

Because both ministers and their environments are changing each minute and each day, self-knowledge is transitory and always incomplete. However, the more self-knowledge ministers acquire, the more appropriate, constructive, and expeditious their behavior will be. The more inaccurate the map, the more inappropriate, destructive, and wasteful their behavior will be.

The following four dimensions of the self are particularly relevant to a minister's effective functioning: one's strengths; weaknesses; motives for acting; and social behavior or impressions.

It is important to recognize one's strong points and to use them to the advantage of oneself and others. Some ministers are unaware of their strengths, and, like a carpenter who is unaware of the tools available, such ministers unnecessarily function at less than optimal levels.

Maybe one of a minister's strengths is the presence of a clear view of reality which can see through tangential issues to the heart of a problem or a situation. Perhaps a minister is capable of great empathy and relates easily with people who are experiencing hurts, fears, angers, or guilts. A minister may have a sound spirituality that enables him or her to place events in a spiritual perspective and to share this perspective in a way that encourages and heals others.

Effective ministers do not mechanically use their strengths as a surgeon uses surgical instruments. But they are aware of their strengths and do not hesitate to capitalize on them when they are most needed or when nothing else seems to be helpful at a particular time.

Besides being aware of their strengths, ministers do well to pay attention to their weaknesses. Ministers who are oblivious to their weaknesses will make the same mistakes over and over again, damaging themselves and others in the process. A minister may tend to be impatient and sometimes treat people as intruders. Instead of asking, "What can *I* do for you?" such a minister asks, "What do *you* want?" Sometimes a minister may tend to use and manipulate people, employing the justification that it is for their own good, when it is actually for the minister's good. Maybe a minister unintentionally harbors biases toward members of the same sex or the opposite sex, toward certain races, classes of people, or religious denominations, or toward certain problems.

Ministers who are unaware of these weaknesses become blunted instruments of the Lord. If they can admit their weaknesses to themselves and to others, they have a good chance to control them, work on them, and ultimately reduce them or even turn them into strengths.

If ministers want to grow in self-knowledge, they have to recognize the motives behind their actions. It is not unusual for people to be unaware of their reasons for making certain decisions or for behaving in certain ways. As human beings, we typically are aware of motives that cause us to feel good about ourselves and unaware of those that create anxiety. When we are aware of some of our motives but unaware of others, we become virtually two people, one of whom is a stranger to the other. This can cause significant confusion and damage to ourselves and others.

For example, a minister chooses to work in an inner-city parish. The minister's choice may be based on the conscious motivation that the poor and oppressed need her more than do middle-class or wealthy people. However, the minister's unconscious motivation is that she expects to receive more appreciation from the inner-city people and be viewed by others as dedicated and strong. When, after a short time, it becomes clear to her that she is actually receiving less appreciation than she did from other people and that people view her no differently than they did before — or perhaps that they view her as foolish — the minister's motivation weakens considerably. Soon she experiences frustration and discouragement and blames her reactions on an unchangeable social system. This allows her to leave the inner-city ministry without ever coming to grips with her deeper motives. Even though the minister blames others for the situation, abandoning this ministry is not good for her: it leaves her experiencing a sense of failure. Nor is the leaving good for the people: the minister was just beginning to develop a reputation as someone who genuinely cared about them, and when she left, the people perceived her as deserting them.

Commonly, hidden motives deal with the needs to acquire power, prestige, attention, romance, control, and the needs to be perceived as competent, holy, intelligent, attractive, clever, successful. None of these motives is inherently problematic; each becomes so only when it is disguised by other motives that appear more acceptable to the person and others.

It is important for ministers to be aware of their social behavior, that is, the impressions that they are giving people. Unfortunately, the impressions we give are not always what we think they are or would like them to be. For example, a minister thinks he gives the impression of being concerned and friendly as he greets people after services. But his artificial smile and his superficial and overplayed attempts to be friendly give the impression of a politician trying to win votes from people about whom he could not care less. So, while his fantasy is that people are admiring his friendliness, they are actually commenting on his phoniness.

Another minister believes that she is impressing people with her knowledge of psychology and theology. Her pedantic style, name-dropping, and unnecessary use of abstract terms actually leave the impression that she is insecure and intellectually narcissistic.

Ministers should give good impressions, but the good impressions should flow spontaneously from their goodness and not be manufactured by the need to be different than they really are. When ministers receive feedback that the impressions they are giving people are unhelpful, they can attempt to discover who they are trying to be that they are not, and they can seek a constructive resolution to the discrepancy.

Self-Esteem and Its Qualities

The second aspect of a healthy sense of self is self-esteem. Self-esteem does not mean pride or narcissism. It simply means that ministers with self-esteem treat themselves as they treat others whom they esteem, that is, with kindness and respect. They also expect to be treated in helpful ways, or at least in ways that do not unduly impair their effectiveness, freedom, or happiness. Ministers who possess at least adequate self-esteem share the following qualities: they have self-respect; they like themselves; they stand up for themselves; and they treat themselves well.

The first quality flowing from self-esteem is self-respect. Self-respect, in turn, helps ministers to communicate clearly who they are without equivocating on their beliefs, feelings, or values. Self-respecting ministers are themselves at all times, and except for superficial differences, they are not more themselves in one situation and less themselves in another. They do not overidentify with the role of minister, wearing it like a cloak to hide their insecurities, inadequacies, ignorance, or doubts. They operate on the principle, "This is who I am right now. I hope you like it, but if you don't, I'd rather be disliked for who I am than liked for who I am not."

Ministers who lack self-esteem do not respect and/or like who they are, either because they distort their goodness through a negative lens of unrealistic expectations and false beliefs, or because they have in ways that do not merit respect and esteem. These ministers represent themselves in ways that are unclear, confusing, and contradictory because they need to hide behind smokescreens. They are chameleon-like, changing color with the psychological and theological terrain. They are one person in the presence of an authority, a second in the presence of friends, a third with family, a fourth with their congregation, a fifth with other ministers, and a sixth when they are alone. They are influenced by powerful and dramatic people, whose mannerisms and values they assume, forsaking their own selves in the process.

Besides possessing self-respect, ministers with self-esteem like themselves. This leads them to appreciate being who they are, to enjoy spending time with themselves, and to enjoy sharing themselves with others.

Ministers who lack adequate self-esteem are basically dissatisfied with themselves and, deep down, wish they were someone else, someone more attractive, intelligent, admired, popular, powerful, or successful. They continually strive after these qualities and/or pretend to themselves and others that they possess them. This causes a continuing state of unrest, the reverberations of which affect the people around them.

Ministers who lack adequate self-esteem seldom enjoy being by themselves. They need to be preoccupied with people and projects so that they do not have to spend time with someone they dislike and find boring, namely, themselves.

Ministers who lack adequate self-esteem are reluctant to share themselves with people because they fear that others will see them as they see themselves and reject them, as they have rejected themselves. As a result, they remain psychologically distant from others, or they place a transparent shield around their hearts, leading people to believe that they are approachable when, in fact, sooner or later it will become obvious that they are not.

Ministers with self-esteem possess a third important quality: they stand up for themselves. They do not allow others to treat them unjustly, to restrict their freedom unduly, or to manipulate them into behaving in ways that are inconsistent with who they are. They see to it that they get what they deserve and that they are allowed to exercise a reasonable degree of free choice. They do not allow themselves to be pressured into behaviors, relationships, or situations that are inimical to their psychological and spiritual well-being.

Ministers who lack self-esteem allow themselves to be ignored and passed over, or to be overburdened when it is inappropriate and destructive. They allow themselves to be imprisoned by the inordinate needs and expectations of others and to be intimidated into behaviors, decisions, and projects for which they are unmotivated and ill-suited. As a result, they feel even lower self-esteem, which creates an endless vicious cycle.

Finally, ministers with self-esteem treat themselves well. This means that they care for themselves as they would care for anyone they like and respect. Their work schedule is reasonable; that is, they do not overwork and sap their energy, effectiveness, and joy; nor do they underwork and feel lethargic, bored, or purposeless. They assiduously avoid relationships and situations that are inordinately depleting and damaging. When it becomes clear that they are in a relationship or a situation in which they are being treated as a scapegoat, a slave, a punching bag, a martyr, a bodyguard, a baby-sitter, or a referee, they disengage themselves, regardless of what others think about them. They have no need to be a victim of anyone or anything.

Such ministers allow themselves adequate leisure time so that they can relax, introspect, enjoy, and rejuvenate themselves. Leisure time is given a high priority, and it is not viewed as something tagged on to the end of the day or the week if there is no other work to do. They confine the majority of their energies, thoughts, and feelings to the present, refusing to mourn the past or fret over the future. Each day is an amorphous piece of clay that they can sculpt to the best advantage for themselves and others.

Ministers with self-esteem keep their emotional state clear. Each significant emotion is acknowledged and expressed spontaneously and appropriately. As a result, by the end of the workday, they are sufficiently buoyant and can enjoy the second half of their day. Ministers with less self-esteem hesitate to express their feelings for fear of losing what limited self-esteem they have. They bottle up their feelings of hurt, anger, fear, and frustration, which adds excess weight to their psyche, body, and soul. They collapse at the end of the workday, ruing all the opportunities they had to change things simply by expressing their feelings. They tell anyone who will listen what they *should* have said, what they *could* have done, what they *felt like* saying. Their unexpressed feelings curdle within them and turn sour, causing them to begin each new day with a larger handicap.

Ministers with self-esteem treat themselves well by making decisions based on the best information available, realizing that a certain percentage of their decisions will turn out less well than they hoped. After they make the decision, they leave it and move on to the next challenge. They do not torture themselves (and others) with indecision, confusion, needless worry, second-guessing, and rumination.

They walk into relationships and situations with their heads up, choosing how they will get involved and for how long. They do not allow themselves to get caught in the wake of other people's needs, getting swept into situations by currents that were too subtle for them to see or too powerful for them to resist. They rarely find themselves lamenting, "How did I get myself into this mess?" or " I knew this wasn't a good idea."

Ministers with self-esteem possess a healthy sense of self-discipline, which frees them to function well. They structure their day and use it well. They do not have long periods of useless time; nor do they over-schedule their day, having to leave appointments early only to get to the next appointment late. They eat, drink, and sleep in moderation, refusing to punish their bodies with excess weight or substances that damage tissues or impair thinking. They get an adequate amount of exercise and keep in reasonably good shape so that their bodies will continue to be strong encasements for their psyches and souls.

Self-Actualization

The third aspect of the healthy self is the ability for self-actualization. This means that effective ministers are self-motivated, self-directing, self-confident, and self-sustaining.

Self-motivating means that ministers must possess intrinsic motivation; that is, they must be self-starters. They must know what they have to do on any particular day, and then do it. Intrinsic motivation is the opposite of both extrinsic motivation and no motivation. Extrinsic motivation means that a minister does not make any significant decisions or take any meaningful action until pressured by others to do so. This causes frustration in other people and resentment in the minister. No motivation means that a minister's laziness, insecurities, fears, frustrations, and resentments have short-circuited his or her motivation, leaving him or her immobilized. This creates dullness or helplessness in the minister and frustration and withdrawal in other people.

The self-actualized minister is also self-directing. This means that psychologically healthy ministers basically make and carry out their own decisions. They examine each important situation with reasonable care, scrutinize the relevant issues, consult with others, make their decision, and accept the responsibility for the consequences.

Therefore, self-actualized and self-directing ministers must also possess reasonable self-confidence, that is, confidence in their intuitions, perceptions, judgments, and decisions. This enables ministers to assert themselves, sharing their ideas, feelings, and values in a clear and forthright manner. Self-confidence does not mean that ministers are confident that they are always correct. It simply means that they are confident that what they say is generally worth considering and will help clarify situations. Such ministers recognize that they will not always be on target, but they are willing at least to illuminate the target with their input.

There are two ways in which ministers can experience difficulty with self-confidence. The first is to believe that they are always, or almost always, correct. Paradoxically, this belief indicates a lack of self-confidence, which, in turn, prevents ministers from seeing their imperfections and taking appropriate corrective action. The second difficulty is that these ministers may not move or progress until they possess absolute moral certitude. Since they rarely, if ever, feel so certain, they remain reticent on anything but the most superficial issues. Both difficulties have the same negative side effects: they render ministers useless as catalysts who could create illumination, and they prevent ministers from being sought after by people who need someone off whom to deflect concerns.

Finally, self-actualized ministers are self-sustaining. This means that ministers must sustain themselves without over-relying on others for their survival. Ministers need to be capable of meeting their own needs for security, freedom, success, justice, stimulation, and leisure.

With regard to interpersonal needs, self-actualized ministers see to it that they relate to people socially (in contrast to pastorally) who are able and willing to participate in mutually fulfilling relationships; that is, to those who are willing to give and receive affection, to trust and be trusted, to give freedom and accept it, to give joy and accept it, to give honesty and receive it.

Sometimes ministers confuse being self-sustaining with being self-sufficient, that is, needing no one else for growth and happiness. This confusion can lead ministers into three problem areas. The first problem is that they may live a half life by depriving themselves of the growth and the joy of getting interpersonal needs met. As a result, these ministers go through life functioning on only half of their psychological and theological cylinders, and they are often unaware of their retardation.

A second problem is that these ministers may experience a deep-seated loneliness, the pain of which they may try to anesthetize with work, prayer, avocations, food, drink, sex, or drugs. However, neither the pain nor its source is ever completely exorcised, and thus never really dealt with.

A third problem with confusing self-sustenance with self-sufficiency is that seemingly self-sufficient ministers might convey the message that they need no one. This causes people to be disinterested in them and remain distant, which, in turn, impairs the minister's apostolic functions.

Some ministers may lack self-sustenance altogether. They may be unwilling or incapable of foraging for themselves; hence they are almost totally reliant on others for nourishment. This dependency places them in a perilously vulnerable position: when they please others, they get fed, but when they displease others, they starve. In order to survive, these ministers must cater to the needs, values, and whims of others, even at the sacrifice of their overall well-being. These ministers are like people who voluntarily hand over their lives to gain simple food and shelter.

Self-Fulfillment

The fourth aspect of a healthy sense of self is self-fulfillment. Just as ministers have physical appetites, they also have psychological appetites. The more psychosocial needs they get met, the more they grow in psychological strength. When ministers fail to get their needs met adequately, three conditions can result: psychological malnutrition, psychological semi-starvation, and psychological starvation.

Psychological malnutrition results when a minister is getting some needs met, but not enough to remain healthy. Some common symptoms of psychological anemia are inordinate discouragement, irritability, confusion, indecision, frustration, hurts, resentment, guilt, cynicism, jealously, forgetfulness, procrastination, or distractibility.

Psychological semi-starvation results when a minister is getting no important needs met to any meaningful degree. Some typical semi-starvation symptoms are clinical depression, anxiety reactions, phobias, obsessions, compulsions, alcoholism, depersonalization, drug abuse, sexual disorders, or psychophysiological reactions (tension headaches, peptic ulcers, compulsive eating, frequent colds, insomnia, high blood pressure, psychogenic menstrual disorders, etc.).

Psychological starvation results from a minister not getting important needs met over a prolonged period of time. Some common starvation symptoms are acute disorientation, serious mood disorders (manic and depressive disorders), schizophrenic disorders, and paranoid reactions.

Most, if not all, ministers require the following "self" needs to be fulfilled in order to minister effectively.

Healthy ministers need:

• *To have affection.* They need to have one or more people need, appreciate, affirm, trust, and support them. They need to have people pay attention to them, demonstrate warmth, tenderness, and empathy, perceive them as special, and love them.

• *To give affection.* This is an underrated need, but one that is as important as receiving affection. It consists of behaving in ways that allow one or more people to feel loved, understood, appreciated, treasured, special, secure, worthwhile, joyful, free to be themselves, and loved.

• *To exercise freedom.* Although ministers realize that reality imposes some unavoidable restrictions, ministers remain unfulfilled — and thus unhealthy — unless they are allowed freedoms such as the following: to pick their friends; to decide the direction of their important decisions; to judge when they will or will not make sacrifices; to determine what their lifestyle will or will not be; to select what professional and religious values they will espouse or eschew; to resolve how long they will stay in a relationship or a situation and when they will leave it; and to choose to whom they do or do not owe loyalty.

• *To experience stimulation.* Although a certain amount of routine is inevitable in life, ministers must see to it that they have a sufficient degree of variety, change, newness, and freshness in their lives. Thus, they should refuse to be stifled by avoidable routine in their jobs, relationships, or life in general.

• *To feel a sense of accomplishment.* While healthy ministers understand that they cannot always see all the fruits of the labors, they make sure that they are able to see some positive results and tangible rewards of their efforts and endeavors in their occupations of personal lives. This helps ministers feel that who they are and what they are doing are worthwhile.

• *To have solitude.* Privacy and peace and quite enable ministers to remain in touch with themselves, to relax, think, pray, or just quietly be.

• *To be treated justly.* While ministers should realize that they are not immune to injustice, they also need to be afforded the respect, freedom, support, recognition, and rewards that they deserve in important relationships and situations.

• *To have hope.* They need to see a light at the end of the tunnel. At some perceivable point in the future, ministers must have the hope to experience a reasonable degree of success or relief from distress.

• *To have a purpose in their lives.* Ministers need a value, a philosophy, or a theology that ties their days, endeavors, joys, and sufferings into one meaningful theme that serves as a frame of reference, a source of encouragement, and an ultimate goal.

• *To experience joy for self-fulfillment.* While healthy ministers realize that life is often difficult and sometimes almost impossible, they also see to it that they experience a reasonable amount of joy. They experience joy from a variety of areas and enterprises: doing a good job, reading, writing, relaxing, athletics, music, art, nature, exercise, social activities, looking attractive, prayer, and relationships.

These "self" (psychosocial) needs are common in our culture and probably in modern cultures. They seem to stem from a combination of biological predisposition and learning. These needs differ in intensity from one person to another, and even within the same person at different times, much the same as do physical needs. Like anyone else, ministers can go about getting these needs met consciously or unconsciously. A minister may consciously decide he needs some joy in his life, so he takes the day off to play tennis, walk along the seashore, or visit a dear friend. Or, without consciously knowing why, a minister may decide it is time to disengage herself from a relationship or a job that has been subtly and gradually usurping her freedom. Both decisions — conscious and unconscious — fulfill the minister's need for joy in life.

Unfortunately, because deprivation in psychosocial needs does not register the clear warning signals that physical need deprivation does, ministers can go for prolonged periods of time depriving themselves of fulfillment in one or more critical areas. The same minister who would never miss a meal or a night's sleep may go for months or even years without getting his or her need for affection, freedom, stimulation, or joy adequately met. Meanwhile the minister wonders why he or she is suffering the psychological hunger pains of fatigue, irritability, illness, anxiety, forgetfulness, depression, cynicism, hopelessness, or spiritual desolation.

It is also important to realize that simply because a minister is in a situation where she "should" be getting her needs met, it does not necessarily mean that they are being met. The minister may have a family or live with a religious community, but the people in her life may not be willing to meet or capable of meeting many of her needs with any degree of consistency. Even if they may be willing to meet and capable of meeting her needs, her unresolved fears, resentments, or guilts may keep her from accepting their love, freedom, or joy.

It is necessary for ministers to understand what their specific needs are, how important each is at any given time, and how he or she plans on getting them met with reasonable consistency. Just as ministers need to eat and sleep each day, they need to get at least some of their needs met each day. It is not sufficient to set aside two weeks a year to relax or four days a year to experience joy.

It is important that ministers *see to it* that *they* get their needs met; that is, that they do not wait passively to be fed by others. Psychologically vibrant ministers arrange their time, work, relationships, and prayer so that most days are at least reasonably, if not maximally, fulfilling. Ministers who suffer from psychological malnutrition typically protest that, due to the way *their life* is *arranged*, they cannot possibly get their needs met adequately. These same ministers would never allow others to arrange their days so that they did not eat or sleep. Sometimes it takes professional help — and in some cases a great deal of help — to get a minister to the point where he or she will assume personal responsibility for his or her psychological diet and nourishment.

Unfortunately, like any one else, ministers may be unaware of crucial needs within themselves, either because the needs have never been primed or because the minister has repressed the need. A minister who has seldom or never experienced true love may be unaware of his need for love. This need may lie dormant throughout life, or become primed only later in life. Again, a minister may repress the need for love because she realizes, at least subconsciously, that if she allows it to surface, it will create great anxiety. On some level the minister knows that if it surfaces but is not met, she will experience great loneliness, which she does not wish to do. If she attempts to reach out to people for love, she may become overly dependent on someone, and thus lose her freedom, or risk rejection. Unconsciously, the minister has decided to let sleeping dogs lie.

Finally, it is important that ministers do not perceive the concept of need fulfillment as selfish or self-indulgent, any more than they view eating three meals a day or sleeping eight hours a night as selfish or self-indulgent. Ministers who do not see to it that their psychosocial needs are met reasonably well each day will be of no better use to themselves or others than if they were to skip a meal or two each day. To the extent that ministers are not psychosocially fulfilled, they cannot be spiritually healthy, nor can they adequately fulfill the psychosocial and spiritual needs of others. Ministers cannot give what they do not have.

In summary, the self of the minister is basic to who he or she is. It is the minister's motor, steering mechanism, and brake. A healthy self provides the minister with good energy, with good steering that allows the minister with good energy, with good steering that allows the minister to stay on the road, and with good brakes for slowing down and stopping when it is appropriate. A less healthy self gives the minister too much or too little energy, poor steering (making it difficult to stay on the road), and defective brakes (causing the minister to slow down and stop when he or she should not or fail to stop when he or she should).

Like an automobile, the self requires continual maintenance. The effects of poor maintenance on the self are the same as on an automobile: sooner or later the minister sputters to a stop, blows up, crashes into something, or runs over people.

Qualities of Effective Pastoral Ministers

The term *pastoral*, as it is used in this essay, denotes a minister's ability to relate with people in ways that are personal, caring, and compassionate, and which, in turn, evoke feelings of trust, comfort, and respect from people. Ministers cannot always be pastoral, any more than they can always be competent or effective. Ministers are only human and cannot control all the factors in every situation. However, ministers can work toward becoming more pastoral, competent, and effective in an increasing number of situations with increasingly different kinds of people.

If the minister is psychologically healthy, then he or she is more apt to be pastorally effective. This section will discuss several qualities that effective pastoral ministers seem to share. Each of these qualities is on a continuum; that is, each can be possessed to degrees that are miniscule, moderate, extensive, or not possessed at all.

It is helpful for ministers not only to recognize what these qualities are but also to understand why they are important and what are the effects when ministers lack these qualities.

A Healthy Spirituality

The first quality that effective pastoral ministers share is a healthy and vibrant spirituality. This means possessing two things: an active prayer life and an assimilated theology.

Effective pastoral ministers have an active prayer life that consists of daily communication with God through talking, meditating, contemplating, and participating in liturgies. Ministers may not substitute good works for prayer any more than a good spouse may substitute hard work for loving communication. If good works remain detached from prayer over a period of time, they can lose their originating purpose, become rote and humanitarian instead of spontaneous and Christian.

The prayer of pastoral ministers cannot simply be a routine performed as part of ministerial self-identity or a duty performed to avoid feeling guilty. Prayer must be engaged in with the same affection, joy, and faithfulness as communication between loving spouses.

Pastoral ministers have a *prayer life*; nonpastoral ministers *say prayers*, and this represents all the difference in the world. Ministers who just "say" prayers separate their prayer from the rest of the day. After their morning prayers, their behaviors does not differ from anyone's else's, except that they may have a different vocabulary, using words like God, Christ, Church, love, law, and sin. A prayer "life" is much more than saying prayers; it is a theme that permeates daily behaviors in significant, observable ways.

Ministers who have a prayer life are more patient, empathetic, courageous, just, and freeing. They rarely find themselves destructively judging people, because they understand that not everyone has had love and justice in their lives. They seldom lack the courage to stand up to any person or institution which is functioning in ways that are detrimental to others. It is very untypical of them to treat people unjustly, that is, to use them, to be dishonest with them, and to refuse to affirm them when it would be appropriate to do so. They do not capture people with indoctrination, but free them with education. They view Jesus as a good friend whom they want to introduce to their other good friends. They do not fear God, or introduce God to people as one introduces the new foreman on the job.

Effective pastoral ministers also have an assimilated theology (in contrast to having virtually no theology or one that is not assimilated). A minister can be very religious but have no theology that ties together and makes sense out of his or her religious behaviors and teaching. This situation is analogous to a college professor who teaches psychology but has no underlying philosophy that affords direction, substance, and meaning to his individual lectures.

A nonassimilated theology means that a person has studied theology, perhaps has a doctorate in theology, but has not assimilated it into his or her life. Such people are like a person who is a psychologist from nine o'clock to five o'clock but acts quite differently the rest of the time. In other words, their knowledge has not become assimilated into their beings; it has become stuck in their intellects and has not flowed into their hearts and souls. Such ministers may be able to quote Christ, Aquinas, Augustine, Calvin, Francis, Dominic, Luther, Ignatius, and Wesley, but they have not been able to capture the spirit of these figures in their daily behavior.

Ministers with an assimilated theology sift it through other, God-given sources of enlightenment, such as psychology, the physical sciences, sociology, anthropology, philosophy, and history. In this way, their theology takes on a depth and an expanse that allows them to grow in all directions — not just vertically — and allows them to have a fuller appreciation of, and empathy toward, the people and the world that God created.

Saying that effective pastoral ministers have an assimilated theology does not mean that they have a private one that has become disconnected from the mainstream of sound theological thought. It simply means that pastoral ministers have a theology that has become *them* and is worn, not like an ill-fitting cloak borrowed from some other person or institution, but like a tailored suit that must be continually altered to fit their ongoing growth.

Helpful Motivation

The second quality shared by effective pastoral ministers is that of helpful motivation. Motives flow from needs and move people to act or not to act. Unfortunately, motives are not always conscious. Therefore, people can honestly think, feel, and say that they are acting for one reason, when, in fact, they are acting for a very different one. The concurrent problems that this discrepancy causes are more readily observed by others than by the person acting. In reality, however, it is unusual for a motive to be absolutely pure. Most motives are two-dimensional; that is, they flow from both altruistic and self-centered needs. Depending upon a motive's "need" source, this two-dimensionality can be helpful or unhelpful in ministry. Ministerial motives arising out of needs for affection, accomplishment, correctness, and power may serve to demonstrate this dichotomy.

The need to give affection motivates helpful behavior when the affection promotes growth in others and causes joy in oneself. Ministers who share affection in ways that cause people to become more accepting and loving of themselves, more free and courageous, and more accepting and loving of others, are being helpful. The fact that ministers feel good because they are instrumental in this growth is healthy and good.

Problems can occur,however, when ministers give affection as an investment in order to seduce people into dependent relationships, to convert them to the minister's religious beliefs, to win their affection, or to own and control them. Giving this type of affection is unhelpful and quite possibly damaging.

The need to receive affection is natural and good. Ministers need as much affection (attention, affirmation, intimacy) as anyone else. However, receiving affection as a goal is best left to the minister's personal life; that is, the minister should seek affection from his or her family, friends, and colleagues. When ministers consciously or unconsciously seek to be liked by the people they serve, three problems arise. First, as long as ministers focus on receiving affection, their attention cannot be adequately focused on the people to whom they are supposed to be ministering. Second, when ministers need to be liked more than they need to have integrity, they are vulnerable to the pressures, manipulations, or whims of people, all of which may be inappropriate or damaging. Third, through the process of natural selection, such ministers tend to attract mutually needy people and exclude the psychologically healthy people that every parish so desperately needs.

The need to feel a sense of accomplishment (achievement, success) motivates helpful behavior when it causes a minister to work and relate in ways that cause others to become closer to Jesus, themselves, and one another. If, in the process, ministers feel a personal sense of accomplishment, they should enjoy it and use it to refuel their efforts.

The need to feel a sense of accomplishment can become problematic, however, when it mostly serves the minister's needs for success, praise, and promotion to a more prestigious status. When this is the case, the people become pawns. Sooner or later, they realize the truth of the situation, and become resentful and disinclined to get involved in future church affairs.

The need to feel special can motivate facilitative behavior when it causes a minister to grow in ways that will increase his or her unique personality, gifts, and values. As the minister grows in this direction, he or she becomes a fuller person and helps others actualize their potential.

The need to be special can create tension, however, when it subtly evolves into a need to feel superior to others; that is, to feel intellectually brighter, morally superior, and spiritually closer to God. This motive will be reflected in the minister's demeanor and will eventually drive people away.

The need to be correct can motivate healthy behavior in ministers when it moves them to become knowledgeable about religion, the Church, and human behavior. The more knowledge they possess, the more effective they can be as religious educators.

The need to be correct can be counterproductive, however, when ministers believe that everything they think is true actually is true, when they cannot tolerate ideas that differ from theirs, and when they cannot admit that they have been in error. When these situations occur, the ministers, as ambassadors of the Church, place it in an incredible light.

Finally, the need to have power can motivate effective behavior in ministers when it causes them to bring about personal, social, and theological change. Positive changes are necessary if the Church and society are to survive and flourish.

The need to be powerful can create difficulties, however, when ministers need to take charge of everything in which they are interested. This motive communicates to people that the minister is the only one who can do things correctly, reduces people to sheep rather than ministers in their own right, and deprives people of considering alternate and, perhaps, more effective ways of accomplishing their goals.

Absolute Honesty

The third quality of effective pastoral ministers is absolute honesty. If the Church, through its ministers, is not scrupulously honest, it is no different than any secular institution, except that by pretending to be better (i.e., more honest), it becomes more pernicious than most secular institutions. To possess the quality of honesty, pastoral ministers must conscientiously avoid rationalizations which allow them to ignore, deny, temper, or distort what they know or believe to be true, even when it would be to their temporary advantage to do so.

Honesty means much more than simply not lying to people. It means that pastoral ministers:

> • tell the whole truth, refusing to hedge in the interests of reducing anxiety in themselves or others;

> • disseminate information accurately, without overplaying or underplaying it to make a point or teach a lesson, no matter how "Christian" the point of the lesson;

> • tell others the reasons for asking them to resign, without resorting to lies or half-truths as a way of being "Christian";

> • inform the people about financial, political, or ecclesiastical decisions and matters which they have the right to know, without resorting to the well-worn rationalization, "What the people don't know won't hurt them";

• disagree, either publicly or privately, with people who espouse beliefs that run contrary to Christian values, even at the risk of losing respect, support, or friends;

• communicate to authority when they cannot follow a particular teaching or directive, even when it would be more political to be silent;

• choose members for consultative groups (schools or parish boards, boards of directors, etc.) based on the members' competence and not on their willingness to go along with the minister's ideas;

• assign ministers and pastors on the basis of their competence (which includes spirituality) and not simply because it is "their turn," or because there is a slot to fill;

• refuse to teach people that certain acts are inherently sinful when the ministers know full well that an individual's subjective state must be taken into serious consideration when judging the sinfulness of an act;

• refuse to tell half-truths about drugs, sex, or alcohol, even when such dishonesty would motivate people to be more judicious in their behavior;

• refuse to use scriptural passages to buttress their position when exegetes have offered different interpretations that are equally cogent;

• refuse to pretend to know more than they actually do about theology, Scripture, ecclesiology, Church law, psychology, or counseling, even when such pretense would save them embarrassment;

• refuse to tell people that they are better or worse than they are in an effort to be helpful.

All pastoral ministers must be especially cautious with regard to honesty. They must take special care not to slip into a skewed logic that will support dishonesty.

The Lord is good,

I am an instrument of the Lord,

Therefore, everything I do must be good.

Honesty requires strength, courage, humility, and a healthy disregard for advancement and the opinions of others.

Healthy Sensitivity

A fourth quality of effective pastoral ministers is a healthy sensitivity to people and to the nuances of situations. Healthy sensitivity lies at the midpoint between being thin-skinned and thick-skinned.

A thin-skinned minister is easily hurt by the criticisms or oversights of others, and is overburdened by the suffering of others. As a result, these ministers are distracted a good deal of the time by hurt, frustration, resentment, or suffering, which impairs their ability to relate comfortably with others. Moreover, their oversensitivity shows and causes people either to treat them with kid gloves or to stay away from them.

Thick-skinned ministers have a psychological crust to protect themselves from hurt. As a result, they tend to be impervious to the needs and frailties of others and to the emotional climate in social situations. Consequently, they unintentionally hurt people and often behave like a bull in a china shop. Their insensitivity keeps people at a distance and significantly impedes the minister's ability to be pastorally effective.

Sensitivity is important in ministers because people often communicate their deepest concerns and feelings in veiled forms: an almost imperceptible change in a tone of voice, a flinch in a facial expression, a shift in posture, or a tightening of hands. Most meaningful communication is sensed, not heard. For example, a distraught woman says to a minister, "My son Peter got arrested last night for shoplifting. I just don't know what to do with him. I'm at my wit's end." The less sensitive minister, who may hear what the woman is saying but who fails to sense what she is asking, replies, "Well, let me give you the name of a social service agency where I think you can get some help."

A more sensitive minister, perceiving the woman's feelings of fear, frustration, anger, guilt, confusion, and desperation, says, "You look as though you are filled with all kinds of feelings that would be good for you to get out. I would like it if we could talk for a while, and see if we can't help you feel better so that you can make some clear decisions."

The sensitive minister focuses on the woman who is present, not on the son who is absent. After the woman talks for a while, she may perceive things more clearly and optimistically and may feel that someone genuinely cares about her. It is at this point that the minister can offer her some referral sources.

In the same situation, an overly sensitive minister replies, "Oh, my gosh, that's terrible! How could your son have done such a thing! You poor thing, your must feel terrible! Here, let me drive you home, and we'll talk to him together. Then I'll make an appointment to see him tomorrow. Meanwhile, I'll call a couple of people I know and see if I can get him some professional help. But you need some support, too. Why don't we meet tonight after dinner and see if we can't help you pull yourself together?"

The overly sensitive response creates three problems. First, the minister is nearly as upset as the woman, so the blind is leading the blind. Secondly, the minister's anxiety causes the woman to become more anxious. Instead of thinking how best to solve her problem, she is wondering how to extricate herself from the minister. Thirdly, by the time the minister is finished dealing with the woman, the minister will be exhausted and virtually useless for the rest of the day.

Ministers must be cautious with regard to the quality of their sensitivity. Many begin their ministry as very sensitive people, but as they experience daily suffering, criticism, and apathy, they laminate their hearts so that they do not feel as much. They become more businesslike and less empathetic. They say all the right words but lack all the right feelings that are supposed to go with the words. Although the lamination around their hearts protects them from pain, it also protects them from experiencing warmth, love, joy, and beauty, the very experiences that would help them also experience pain without becoming injured.

Gentle Strength

Gentle strength is the fifth quality possessed by effective pastoral ministers. Ministers can be both gentle and strong at the same time. The quality of gentle strength is necessary for effective pastoral ministry for several reasons.

It is important because ministers must stand up for true Christian values in a world, and sometimes (paradoxically) in a Church, that would find other values more diplomatic or expedient. In holding forth these values, ministers risk being scorned and rejected. To decline to proclaim values such as love, justice, freedom, and honesty is weak and nonministerial. At the same time, to proclaim these values in a harsh, intimidating manner is unchristian. Representing Christian values publicly must be done with a gentleness that flows from genuine concern rather than from fear or anger, and with a strength that denotes commitment and conviction.

Gentle strength is important because it is the basis of assertiveness. Gentle strength lies at the midpoint between being unassertive and aggressive. Ministers must be able to present their ideas, feelings, beliefs, and values in straightforward, clear ways; and they must be able to remain steadfast in the face of manipulation, unrealistic expectations, or impossible requests.

Gentle strength is also the basis for resistance to stress. Effective ministers are involved in many areas of responsibility, and this involvement can cause stress, sometimes great stress. Ministers who are gentle but not sufficiently strong may become worn down or bowled over by stress. Ministers who are strong but lack gentleness may be ungentle with themselves, failing to protect themselves from stress, and unable to perceive the internal clues of pending physical or psychological problems.

Gentle strength denotes an ability to be flexible when situations merit it. Unmitigated and unswerving strength is not always a virtue and, in fact, can be a liability in a minister. For example, there are times when moral judgments must take a backseat to gentleness, compassion, and understanding; and there are times when it is appropriate for ministers to accede to the beliefs, the wishes, and the values of others.

On the one hand, ministers must make difficult decisions that cause anxiety or unhappiness in some people. Because effective ministers are strong, they do not shirk making these decisions. On the other hand, because effective ministers are gentle, they are careful to make decisions which reflect sensitivity to the people and the issues involved.

Gentle strength is also necessary for perseverance, a quality that is often called upon in ministry. Because of human nature, ministers are often faced with people and projects that cause them to feel frustrated and, at times, discouraged. However, a gentle strength allows ministers to keep trying to minister in ways that are unabrasive and increasingly fruitful.

Finally, a gentle strength allows ministers to extricate themselves from damaging relationships and unworkable situations. Their strength allows ministers to retreat, even though it will upset others; their gentleness allows them to withdraw in the most painless ways possible.

Ministers who are too gentle may be that way because of their personalities, because they do not want to cause anxiety in themselves or others, or because they view gentleness as a Christian virtue and strength (assertiveness, confrontation) as unchristian, even though there is ample evidence of Christ being equally gentle and strong.

Ministers who are too strong may be that way because of their personalities, because gentleness is viewed as weakness and thus creates anxiety within them, or because they have overidentified with the strength of Christ and underidentified with his gentleness.

Ministers who are too gentle are inclined to be manipulated, non-confrontive of people and situations that should be confronted, and nonassertive. Ministers who are too strong think they can muscle people into Christian behavior with intellectual assaults, emotional tirades, and theological threats. In addition, they are insensitive to people's frailties and to the nuances of delicate situations. This causes others to view such ministers as threats or as objects of derision.

Genuinely Freeing

Being a person who is genuinely freeing is the sixth quality of effective pastoral ministers. Ministers who are genuinely freeing allow others to exercise freedom of will and freedom of choice. Freedom is a basic Christian value. A good deal of Christ's message deals with freeing people from the inappropriate and unhealthy restraints of the law, politics, religious myths, families, social mores, and worship.

In a Christian context, freedom does not mean unbridled freedom; it does not mean that people are free to behave in ways that are destructive; it does not imply that all restraints are inappropriate or unhealthy. Rather, freedom means that people are free to make their choices and decisions within the broader boundaries of justice and love. Effective ministers realize that often there is not just one path to justice and love, and that the path a particular person takes may not be the one the minister would choose. However, when such a situation occurs — and it may occur with some frequency — effective ministers stand by the person and assist him or her in any way in which the ministers feel comfortable; and that assistance does not necessarily imply that the ministers would have taken the same path. Perhaps one of the acid tests of truly pastoral ministers is that they stand by and help a person even when they may not agree with the person's decision.

Pastoral ministers *invite* people to follow them toward Jesus. It is not a casual invitation ("I don't really care if you follow me or not"); but neither is it a direct order ("Follow me to Christ or else you will be doomed"). Ministers understand that many paths lead to the kingdom and that they represent but one of those paths. In addition to the theological reasons for inviting people to follow Christ, there are equally sound psychological ones. A kind yet concerned invitation is far more likely to attract people than is a command performance. Ministers who abide by a "take it or else" approach are likely to repulse people who, in a modern democratic society, generally bolt at being told that they *must* do something, or they will attract a frightened, resentful following, which is not what Christ had in mind.

It seems that ministers who exert their wills on the people rather than allow people to use their own wills are not working as much in the service of Jesus as in the service of themselves.

They have overidentified with their message, and they feel that to reject it is to reject them. Their attempts to convert people to Christ are veiled attempts to convert people to themselves, much as possessive parents are less concerned about their children's welfare than they are concerned about keeping their children dependent upon them.

Pastoral ministers do not use freedom as a manipulative ploy to draw people to them. This very subtle, sometimes unconscious, dynamic happens even when a concerned, loving person uses the offer of freedom to trap people. This dynamic is based on the message, "I'll prove to you how really good and loving I am by giving you complete freedom to leave me in order to follow someone else or to follow your own lights." The hope is that the person will realize how absolutely good, loving, and unselfish the minister is, and will feel even more attracted and indebted to him or her.

True pastoral ministers free people to be absolutely honest with them. People know that they can disagree with their ministers and that they can decline an invitation to work or relate socially with him or her without damaging the relationship. Unfreeing ministers send the message, "I will be hurt or angry if you don't agree with everything I say or do, or if you say no to me." People who receive this message either cater to the minister — even when it may not be in their best interests, and even when it breeds resentment — or they stay away from the minister because they do not want to get trapped.

If ministers feel compelled to bring people to Jesus because they feel they have been mandated by God to do so or because bringing people to Jesus is an integral part of their personal sense of self-worth, they will feel the same intense pressure as does a salesman who must meet quotas and deadlines, and the effect on them is the same. Ministers will become high-pressure salespeople for Christ, treating people like potential customers who must be manipulated, seduced, loved, and threatened into buying the product. If the person refuses to "buy," the minister feels like a failure and makes the person feel foolish or doomed.

Acting this way is both unchristian and ineffective. A more valid, less pressurized attitude would be to view oneself as a tour guide who can lead people to some beautiful places. If people would prefer to launch out on their own, they are freely allowed that option and are always welcome to return to the tour if they choose. In addition, the tour guide (minister) does not define his or her worth by *how many* people he or she gets to sign up for the tour, but by how he or she treats people, whether or not they choose to follow him or her.

Unconditionally Present

The quality of being unconditionally present to people means that whatever decisions people make and however far from the kingdom their paths wander, the effective pastoral minister will always be at their side, attempting to shed light and bring assistance.

It does not mean that ministers must unconditionally love all people, because this seems to be terribly unrealistic, at least by my definition of love. But ministers can be always present, ready to help people in all ways but those that would cause people to stray from goodness.

Ministers shed the light of faith, and when people get lost despite the light, ministers go out and look for them. Ministers also realize that there are many paths that lead to the kingdom, and the fact that a person chooses an unpopular one does not necessarily mean that he or she is less of a Christian.

Ministers are in a particularly good position to be unconditionally present to people because it is often very difficult for loved ones to do so with a child, a spouse, a parent, or a close friend who makes choices or behaves in ways that are perceived as wrong, destructive, selfish, or sinful. Loved ones are often so hurt, threatened, confused, or guilty about the person's behavior that they must disassociate themselves from the person to avoid being overcome by anguish. A minister, who is typically less emotionally involved in the situation, is freer to stand by the person, just as the physician is better able to treat a child than is the child's parent.

To be able to be present unconditionally, ministers must separate themselves from the "rock throwers," that is, from those Christians who, because of their own unresolved conflicts, throw rocks at sinners or at people whom they perceive to be sinners. Ministers cannot be in a position of throwing rocks and then rushing to stem the bleeding caused by the very rocks that they and their fellow Christians have thrown. By the same token, ministers must be willing to get hit by some rocks as they minister to the victims of the rock throwers.

This is not easy — to be stoned for no other reason than that one is helping a fallen Christian who cannot get up because other Christians are pelting him or her with rocks. Being a rock thrower is easy. It is easy to denounce abortion. It is much more difficult to help a woman who has decided to have an abortion through the abortion and to help her live the rest of her life as fully as she can.

It is easy to denounce premarital sex. It is much more challenging to help a young woman who is pregnant outside of marriage and the boy who has fathered the child live through and after this difficult period in the most effective, helpful, and Christian way.

It is easy to denounce divorce. It is much more arduous to help people live and perhaps even grow through a divorce so that they can become fuller people and more committed Christians.

It is easy to denounce homosexuals. It is much more difficult to help a homosexual to strive to become a better Christian, despite obstacles that fellow Christians place before him or her.

It is easy to denounce people who have left the more established kinds of ministry. It is harder to remain with them, offering the support they sometimes need to pave a different path toward the kingdom.

Toward sinners and people they perceive to be sinners, rock throwers harbor attitudes such as "They should be left to stew in their own juices," or "They made their bed, now let them lie in it," or "They deserve to get their comeuppance." Pastoral ministers do not subscribe to these attitudes.

Ministers have all they can do to be helpful to, and compassionate with, people who are suffering, just as ambulance attendants at an accident have all they can do to treat the victims. And, just as ambulance attendants leave it to the courts to judge who caused the accident, ministers do the psychological and spiritual resuscitation and leave the judging to God.

When the rock throwers return home to the warmth and comfort of their righteousness, the minister remains behind to begin the arduous, unpopular, and sometimes thankless task of being unconditionally present.

Intellectually Competent

Whatever facet of ministry a person is involved in, he or she needs to be competent to carry out its responsibilities. This does not necessarily mean that ministers must be highly educated or possess academic degrees. Some very competent ministers do not possess a good deal of formal education, while some less than competent ministers have the highest academic degrees attainable. Whatever their formal education, competent ministers seem to possess the following qualities.

They possess a breadth of knowledge that covers the area in which they teach. Their knowledge is not inordinately limited by their intelligence, personal biases, aversion to study, insecurity, overconfidence, or laziness.

They do not learn their Christianity by rote and pass it along to others in a parrot-like fashion. They sift the information through a process of critical thinking, discussion, argumentation, and meditation, allowing it to seep from their intellects into their psyches and souls so that it becomes an integral part of them. This process constitutes the critical difference between having knowledge and being knowledgeable.

Competent ministers are intellectually growing. This means that effective ministers continually study and learn. They keep up with the religious literature as conscientiously as physicians, attorneys, and psychologists keep current with the literature in their fields. Ministers are never too experienced, busy, tired, contented, or old to learn a good deal more than they know. They realize that the more they know and understand, the more they can grow and help others grow.

Ministers are intellectually flexible and are willing to try new methodologies in order to increase their effectiveness. They are not anchored to one theory, philosophy, or technique by which they live or die. They recognize that what works with one person or group may be a disaster with another.

Thus, competent ministers are willing to listen to the people's needs and suggestions and to modify their teaching accordingly, rather than having a plan that they foist on people, regardless of whether or not it is suitable for them.

Ministers are intellectually democratic and search everywhere for truth. They read the works and attend the workshops of other denominations. They study other fields, such as psychology, sociology, philosophy, anthropology, and biology, in an attempt to augment and strengthen their understanding of themselves, others, life, and God. They are open to any ideas that are helpful, whether they come from liberals, moderates, or conservatives, from women or men, or from ordained or nonordained people. They do not possess a "private club" mentality, which holds that anyone or anything outside of their group could have nothing worthwhile to offer.

Competent ministers are intellectually creative. Their idea of ministry is to stimulate themselves and others to think for themselves. They do not simply record what they read and hear, then play back the tape for their audiences, who, in turn, replay it for family and friends. Intellectually competent ministers digest what they read and hear, and they modify it with their own ideas, perceptions, and experiences. In one situation, the modification may be to taper what they read and hear, and in another situation, it may be to add to it. In other words, such ministers do not discount the fact that they themselves can be a source of knowledge, and they do not rely solely on others for enlightenment. By the same principle, they stimulate others to think for themselves by questioning, challenging, and encouraging others to add their own wisdom, creating a second force.

Competent ministers are intellectually discerning. They carefully evaluate what they read and hear, and measure it against logic, common sense, objectivity, what others say, and their own experiences. They do not believe something simply because someone in authority proclaimed it, or someone they admire believes it, or someone holy said it. On the other hand, they do not automatically discount something because someone in authority proclaimed it, or someone they don't like believes it, or someone unholy said it. Thus, by the same principle, such ministers are discerning in what they teach and preach, being prudent and careful not to say things that could be easily misconstrued by their audiences. For example, what a minister says to a group of middle-aged adults may be imprudent to say to a group of teenagers, and vice versa.

Competent ministers are intellectually honest. This means that pastoral ministers appreciate the limitations inherent in knowing God. Therefore, they do not pretend to have knowledge about the nature and workings of God that, in reality, no human being possesses or will ever possess. Ministers may possess great faith and hope in God, but they do not confuse this with great knowledge. In their teaching and preaching, they are careful to indicate clearly the differences between theological facts, theories, hypotheses, interpretations, educated guesses, myths, uncertainties, legitimate hopes, and wishful thinking.

Because they recognize the great abyss between limitlessness of God and their own severely limited human intellect, ministers feel completely comfortable admitting theological ignorance, confusion, and doubt. They place their integrity above all else and do not teach and preach precepts or directives with which, in good conscience, they disagree.

Approachability

The ninth, and final, quality of effective pastoral ministers is approachability. It is important that people feel comfortable with, and free to approach, a minister. A minister's effectiveness is in direct proportion to his or her proximity to the people. Ministers can communicate one of the three following messages relevant to approachability:

• "I am someone with whom you can share your being";

• "I am someone you'd want to officiate at your wedding or invite to supper, but not someone with whom you could share your innermost self";

• "I am someone you would prefer to avoid, except when transacting necessary business."

The approachable minister must develop qualities that allow him or her to speak only the first message. Approachable ministers seem to share the following qualities. First of all, they are not afraid to let people come close to them. And when they allow that closeness, they are not afraid that they will become attached to, exploited, trapped, or found wanted by the other person. They have sufficient love in their lives and enough self-control that they will not become attached. They have sufficient strength and assertiveness that they would not allow themselves to be misused. And they have sufficient self-confidence and self-worth that, whether or not they are found wanting, they can handle it with equanimity.

Secondly, approachable ministers are perceived as warm, understanding, and accepting. Warm means gentle and affections, in contrast to rigid and distant. Understanding means that the ministers are able to empathize with people, in contrast to perceiving them as silly, stupid, or weak. Accepting means that ministers invite the other into their lives as he or she is, in contrast to denying entrance until the person meets certain criteria.

Thirdly, approachable ministers *speak with* people; they do not *preach at* them. They are not programmed by theological tapes, but are real, unique, spontaneous people who defy stereotyping. Thus, they do not have pat answers — many times they have no answers — just an informed willingness to help. They do have a sense of humor and humility that helps them keep both themselves and their work in a healthy perspective, which precludes them taking themselves too seriously.

Fourth, approachable ministers recognize the difference between what is real and what is ideal, and they do not act as if the two were synonymous or even very close. Thus, they know the difference between heaven and earth and do not expect mere mortals to think and behave like angels. They are close to God but down-to-earth, so that anyone can understand, challenge, and feel comfortable with them.

Fifth, approachable ministers are well aware of their humanity — of their frailties, weaknesses, and failures. This exquisite awareness of their dark side precludes even the slightest inclination toward pretension, arrogance, or superciliousness, all of which are unbecoming in any person with insight and much less so in a minister. Because they are aware of their humanity, ministers can deal comfortably with the humanity of others without being shocked or repulsed by it. Since these ministers allow their humanity to show, they do not project an idealized image that scares off others.

Finally, approachable ministers balance their intellect and emotions. That is, they do not operate mostly on the basis of thoughts, principles, laws, syllogisms, and deductive or inductive reasoning. Rather, they realize that there is much more to life than law and logic and that few people have been drawn closer to God by an idea, no matter how noble or correct. On the one hand, ministers do not overwork their emotions. They do not allow feelings of love, hope, happiness, or fervor to override the unpleasant aspects of reality in themselves and others. On the other hand, they do not allow feelings of sadness, anger, frustration, or discouragement to override the positive aspects of reality in themselves and others.

Unfortunately, ministers' religious training can sometimes be so concerned with dogma, law, logic, absolutes, moral judgments, and perfection that ministers may evolve from it acting like religious robots. They do all the right things in the wrong ways: they talk to people without communicating with them; they counsel people without helping them; they teach people without educating them; they rub against people without touching them; they love people without liking them; they lead prayers without praying; and they live without life.

Approachable ministers recognize that they are human beings with both intellect and emotions. That combination, though not always synchronized, constitutes a powerful instrument of psychological and spiritual growth for the ministers themselves and for others as well.

Ministers who lack the above pastoral qualities are not good for the soul. Either they are not invited into the souls of people, or if they are, they do damage that could have eternal ramifications. No minister is perfectly pastoral, but it is important for every minister to work continuously toward that goal.

Effective pastoral ministers are good for the soul. They are invited into people's souls and have a strengthening, freeing, and peaceful effect as they work within the depths of the person. Although not everyone needs a physician or a psychologist, everyone needs a *pastoral* minister, whether or not he or she recognizes it.

CHAPTER 7

ON BECOMING A HELPER

Thomas N. Hart

R oman Catholics have been brought up with the idea that there are seven sacraments, each a channel of grace, each, on a more recent presentation of the matter, an encounter with Christ. This is true and important. Each of the seven sacraments is a meeting with God, the deepening of the relationship, an increase in life. The unfortunate byproduct, however, of a concentration on ritual sacraments as the time of the encounter with God is that it diverts attention from all the other encounters and experiences of God's grace, the ones which have no names and come to us unsought and unprepared for. We go to church to find him, and wait for the "real presence" and communion. Our spirituality would be much richer if we realized that these are only some of the ways God meets us. If God is alive and well, interested in his world, and present to it at all times and places, if he is a God who is always disclosing himself and offering himself for relationship, then we may be in a communication situation much more than we usually imagine.

The Second Vatican Council has formally broadened the notion of sacrament in the Church, endorsing an emphasis which has become increasingly dominant in theological reflection. Returning to a notion of sacrament as old as the Fathers of the Church, the council calls attention to the fact that there are two levels of sacramentality more basic than that of the ritual sacraments. Christ is the primordial sacrament. The Church is the next most basic sacrament. Then come the seven ritual sacraments, derivatively.

Christ is a sacrament because he incarnates God and reveals him. "He who sees me sees the Father" (Jn 14:9). Incarnation and sacrament are the same idea: an invisible reality finds a visible embodiment, and what is transcendent comes to us in matter. God is the great mystery beyond our grasp; in Christ, we touch him. We hear his word, feel his care, experience his faithfulness, know his compassion and his mercy. Thus Christ is the primordial sacrament.

> That which was from the beginning, which we have heard, which we have seen with our eyes, which we have looked upon and touched with our hands, the word of life...we proclaim to you (1 Jn 1:1-3).

Next comes the Church. The Church is not a building or a great many buildings. These are places where the Church gathers. The Church is not a hierarchy and a priesthood. These are individuals within the Church who provide an important service. The Church is all God's people. The images employed by Vatican II to set forth the mystery of the Church as the dominant biblical images: People of God, Sheepfold, Body of Christ, Bride of Christ, Branches of the Vine. They are people images, organic, and they are the most original descriptions of the Church we possess. What they point up is a truth we have sometimes forgotten, taking the part (the hierarchy) for the whole: that the Church is the community of all those persons who belong to Christ.

Vatican II calls this community of persons a sacrament (*Constitution on the Church, 1*). The designation may seem odd, but its explanation is found in the basic notion of sacrament already considered. Like Christ, Christians incarnate something and bring it to visibility. What we incarnate is Christ, and that is why we are called the body of Christ. For Jesus of Nazareth is no longer present as an individual on the stage of history, as he was for a limited period of time in the first century. He died, and has undergone transformation into the glorified state. His incarnation in the world now is the Church, all those human beings who have been baptized into him and breathe his Spirit.

Let us be concrete and experiential about this sacramentality of Christians. Why were the slaves who came in off the slave ships to Cartagena in the seventeenth century, sick, lonely, afraid, sometimes near death, so moved when they came into contact with Peter Claver? Because he incarnated the love and ministry of Christ. Why are the dying poor in Calcutta's streets so moved and uplifted by their contact with Mother Teresa and her sisters? Because they incarnate the love and ministry of Christ. Why do we respond as deeply and strongly as we do to our contacts with a really good priest or minister, whether that encounter be ritually sacramental or not? Because his presence, his words, his relation to us so unmistakably carry Christ's own presence and activity. Why do some people say they experience God more profoundly on a beautiful Sunday morning in a backyard brunch with their family than they do in going to church? Why do others testify that a dinner with a close friend over life's important questions is more of a religious experience for them than the Eucharist often is? Is not this too because there is a kind of pervasive sacramentality in the world which bears God to us, so that when we touch the depths of any experience we touch him? Well, is there any more compelling bearer of the holy than the human person made in God's image and likeness in the first place, and, as a Christian, striving to put on Christ? This is the root of the Church's sacramentality.

Here we have the explanation of a very important saying of Jesus:

> Jesus answered then, "Destroy this temple, and in three days I will raise it up"... But he spoke of the temple of his body. When therefore he was raised from the dead, his disciples remembered that he had said this, and they believed the scripture and the word which Jesus has spoken (Jn 2:19-22).

In the Old Testament, the Temple was the holy place, God's own house. This saying of Jesus about destroying it naturally got him into trouble with the religious authorities, and they used it as evidence against him in his trial (Mk 14:58). For by these words he signifies nothing less than a religious revolution. God's temple is no longer a building, but Jesus' body. This is the holy place now, the place of the encounter with God. That might be easy enough for us Christians to accept, believing as we do in the divinity of Christ. But have we adverted sufficiently to the meaning of his body? What is his body? During the life of the historical Jesus, it is his own person. But the passage speaks explicitly of his resurrection. After his resurrection, his body is the church. The early Christians built no churches, but broke bread in their homes (1 Cor 11:17-34). It was in one another that they met, reverenced and served God.

Do you not know that your body is a temple of the Holy Spirit within you, which you have from God? (1 Cor 6:19).

Now you are the body of Christ and individually members of it (1 Cor 12:27).

Truly, I say to you, as you did it to one of these, the least of my brothers or sisters, you did it to me (Mt 25:40).

Saul, Saul, why do you persecute me? (Acts 9:4).

The person who receives you receives me, and the one who receives me receives him who sent me (Mt 10:40).

If we really grasped this sacramentality of the Christian community, it would make an immense difference to our spirituality.

Helper as Sacrament

Now let us look specifically at the helping relationship in the context of the Church. We are social beings; none of us makes it alone. Where the genesis and nurture of our faith are concerned we depend vitally on that community of persons who are grounded in the same faith experience. Though our prayer be often solitary and the responsibility of our life ultimately our own, we do not deal with God in a vacuum, but in the context of a human community. At certain times, especially, we feel the need of someone's help. What do we find when we seek it? Just another human being? No. If the Church is sacramental, if human beings, in the Spirit of Jesus, are the sacrament of God's presence and action in the world, then we meet more than the person whose assistance we seek. The encounter is sacramental. It does not matter whether the helper is ordained or not, or whether the transaction is an officially acknowledged ritual sacrament or not. The invisible is somehow present in the visible.

Out of this comes the helper's most basic self-understanding. Any helping relationship in the context of Christian faith is a mysterious encounter. God is somehow present and at work in it. What the helper is doing goes beyond his or her powers and his or her deliberate intent. He or she does everything possible, uses all available personal resources, thinks and acts as if everything depended on him- or herself. At the same time he or she knows that all of this is just a vehicle for something larger than itself, whose operation is hidden and unsearchable, whose influence goes beyond the means at hand and even the ends sought. The work of the helper is in this respect like the work of the preacher. We know what we say and we know what we mean. But what God may be saying in our words to any given hearer is a matter quite beyond our calculation or control. It makes sometimes for the greatest surprises.

> To him whose power at work in us is able to accomplish more than we could ask or even conceive, to him be glory in the church and in Christ Jesus, now and forever. Amen. (Eph 3:20).

The helper can properly regard him-or herself as making God present to the other in God's concern, compassion, acceptance, support. People need that. God can seem very distant, and oneself very much alone. God may well be believed in, but there is no real experience of him. He is a notion, not a reality perceived. And then comes incarnation. At the hands of someone in a helping role, a person sees flesh and blood on a lot of faith notions. God is real, is present, does care; his word heals, his assurance gives strength, his faithfulness is life. Through the experience of being ministered to by one who shows a genuine personal concern, an acceptance which goes beyond one's deserts, and an affirmation of all that is good in one's life, a person can believe, perhaps for the first time, that God is love and what he is said to have said is true. The helper takes one seriously, and implicitly expresses the confidence that one can take responsibility for one's own life and turn it to some account. This gives the person the exultant feeling that God himself is holding out life as something precious, and offering a person his or her selfhood as a gift and charge of immense value.

The importance of incarnation or sacramentality to our life with God can hardly be overestimated. In the Old Testament, when God called the prophet Samuel as a young boy, Samuel did not know what he was dealing with or how to read the communication. He needed the help of an older man schooled in God's ways to confirm and clarify his vocation (1 Sam 3). The advice the old man, Eli, gave was that Samuel should say, when he felt the Lord calling, "Speak, Lord, your servant is listening." When he did that, the Lord's message came clear to him. Many is the person since who has been confused about the way God was dealing with him or her, and found clarity only in talking it through with someone else who shared the faith and knew something of God's ways.

It is instructive to note how much Jesus uses the sacramental principle in his ministry, particularly where healings are concerned. Over and above the sacrament of his own historical personality, he uses all sorts of material media for the action of God. He lays his hand on the leper (Mk 1:41), puts his fingers into the ears of the deaf and dumb man and touches his tongue and spittle (Mk 7:33), tells the blind man to go wash in the pool of Siloam after he anoints his eyes with clay (Jn 9:7), tells the ten lepers to go show themselves to the priests (Lk 17:14). He can heal at a distance without any apparent instrumentality, but even there it is his word, accepted in faith, that effects the cure (Jn 4:40). Thus it is typically in some sacramental or materially mediated way that Jesus gives new life to individuals. This is God's accommodation to humanity, for we are body-persons. John Henry Newman noted long ago that we are influenced much more by what is concrete and immediate than by what is abstract, even if it is logically reasoned. All religions are aware of it, having their sacred times, sacred places, sacred objects, sacred persons. The sacramental principle is God's way of dealing with us, making the invisible visible, the inaudible audible, the intangible tangible. In a helping relationship in the context of faith, sacramentality is the key to understanding its mysterious efficacy.

Beset with Weakness

This could be misunderstood. The helper somehow embodies the presence of Christ, yet may lack many of the virtues of Christ. The helper's words somehow carry a word of God to the other person, but the helper should never confuse his or her words for those of the Lord. The helper may be able to do quite remarkable things for people, but should never allow him- or herself to be puffed with pride at the ownership of such great power.

Perhaps it is precisely to make such mistakes difficult that God typically gives the helper a profound feeling of inadequacy and personal poverty. The title of Henri Nouwen's book, *Wounded Healer*, perfectly expresses the paradox. Because this is such a common experience, it merits consideration.

We usually think of St. Paul as the epitome of personal strength and self-assurance. Not only does he take strong theological positions and state them with uncompromising boldness; he takes on both the multitudes and the powers that be with indomitable courage. Add to this his testimony of extraordinary religious experiences in his conversion and his visions and revelations, and you have the picture of a man who apparently lies prey to no doubts, and cannot be turned aside from his objectives either by difficulty or penalty. Yet it is this Paul from whom we have the words: "We have this treasure in earthen vessels, to show that the transcendent power belongs to God and not to us" (2 Cor 4:7). It is Paul who writes:

To keep me from being too elated by the abundance of revelations, a thorn was given me in the flesh, a very messenger of Satan, to keep me from being too elated. Three times I besought the Lord about this, that it should leave me; but he said to me, "My grace is sufficient for you, for my power is made perfect in weakness" (2 Cor 12:7-9).

It is not difficult to find ourselves in this portrait. We too have thorns in the flesh, and would love to be without them. They bother us, and often they seem to impede our effectiveness in doing God's work. We often feel our weakness, the fragility of an earthen vessel carrying a treasure on which it has far too vulnerable a hold. Sometimes this becomes quite acute, as people press on us with their many needs, and we search our souls wondering what we shall give to them: "There is a lad here who has five barley loaves and two fish; but what are they among so many?" (Jn 6:9). We can never extricate ourselves from the embarrassing position of fellow struggler, seeker, sufferer. Sometimes our woes seem too great to allow us to look up from them and open ourselves to the pains of another. Well, Paul has apparently felt this too. He describes himself as hanging on by a thread at times:

We are afflicted in every way, but not crushed; perplexed, but not driven to despair; persecuted, but not forsaken; struck down, but not destroyed (2 Cor 4:8-9).

This describes the precarious character of his life and work, but then he goes on to heighten the paradox, and again we find our apostolic experience enshrined in this statement:

...always carrying in the body the death of Jesus, so that the life of Jesus may also be manifested in our bodies. For while we live we are always being given up to death for Jesus' sake, so that the life of Jesus may be manifested in our mortal flesh. So death is at work in us, but life in you (2 Cor 4:10-12).

Death is at work in us, but life in you. The suffering and death of Jesus is not a once-and-for-all event touching only him. It is something all of us participate in over and over in many ways, without its necessarily ever coming to the drama of an actual crucifixion. The mystery at work here, as in the case of Jesus himself, is that the death we die is somehow life-giving for others. It is fruitful, even while it seems to be destroying us. In the midst of our suffering and inadequacy, we mediate something to others that is not our own possession and which we usually cannot even feel passing through our system. We instinctively suppose we should work from strength, handing on to others the riches that are ours. Instead, we often do our best when we operate from weakness and totally empty hands, passing on something we do not possess, producing effects we can in no way explain out of who or how we are. God's economy is bizarre; there is no employment quite as baffling as his. Again Paul speaks of it:

When I came to you, brothers and sisters, I did not come proclaiming to you the testimony of God in lofty words of wisdom. For I decided to know nothing among you except Jesus Christ and him crucified. And I was with you in weakness and in much fear and trembling; and my speech and my message were not in plausible words of wisdom, but in demonstration of the Spirit and of power, that your faith might not rest in the wisdom of human beings but in the power of God (1 Cor 2:1-5).

There is good reason for dwelling this way on our involvement in the paschal mystery even when we are trying to help. For unless we understand it, we will shrink back from agreeing to serve others in a helping capacity, precisely because we so keenly feel weakness, fear and trembling, thorns in the flesh, death in our own mouths. Common sense dictates staying out of other people's lives. But God's is not exactly a common sense economy. The fact is that some of our best preachers have to drag themselves into the pulpit to do it, some of our best consolers dread nothing more than having to go out and be with those who mourn, some of our best prayer leaders pray with heavy hearts, and some of our best counselors and therapists have little sense most of the time that they are doing anything for those who sit before them. They achieve what they achieve because it is not really their achieving. What is asked of them is simply that they be willing, in faith, to present themselves, to go there, to open their mouths and speak what comes out. It would take a lifetime to get ready, and then we wouldn't be ready. Jeremiah said, "Ah, Lord God! Behold, I do not know how to speak, for I am only a youth." But God said to him:

Do not say, "I am only a youth"; for to all to whom I send you you shall go, and whatever I command you you shall speak. Be not afraid of them, for I am with you to deliver you, says the Lord (Jer 1:6-8).

Moses humbly offered the same demurrer, and got the same reply (Ex 3). Paul felt it too, as we have seen, but after the Lord's word to him, he had a kind of conversion experience, acquiesced in the mystery of God's ways, and ended by saying:

I will all the more gladly boast of my weaknesses, that the power of Christ may rest upon me. For the sake of Christ, then, I am content with weaknesses, insults, hardships, persecutions, and calamities; for when I am weak, then I am strong (2 Cor 12:9-10).

The helper is sacrament for the other. Like all sacraments we are inadequate to the reality we flesh forth. We are mere earthen vessels, to show that the amazing power belongs to God and not to us (2 Cor 4:7).

ESTABLISHING AN ORIENTATION

In the preceeding sections we looked at the helping relationship in the context of Christian faith. Now let us focus on the role of the helper and try to come to a more exact notion of what he or she is trying to do. A relationship can come to grief if we do not understand what we are doing. We ourselves can come to grief if we ask the impossible of ourselves. So let us attempt a role description, first setting forth what the helping role is, then clarifying it further by stating what it is not.

What It Is...

1. To Listen

A helper is, in the first instance, one who agrees to listen. Anything else that may happen in the relationship will derive from this. Listening to another may not seem like much, but its effect happens to be very therapeutic. Everyone yearns to be heard. But so many cannot find anyone who will listen, or do not trust most people to be able to handle what they really need to say. So they come to you.

Listening is not always easy. It takes time, and the time might be inconvenient besides. It demands really being there for the other during that period, further present and attentive, one's own needs and concerns set aside. This is exacting. Listening might mean being afflicted with the most profound sense of helplessness, having the springs of sorrow touched, seeing one's dearest convictions called painfully into question by the experience and testimony of another. The person may not be attractive, might be telling a dull and too oft repeated tale, might be making mountains out of molehills, might be demanding and even manipulative. These are the hazards. Nevertheless there comes to me a human being whom God created and loves. There comes a sister or brother for whom Christ died (Rm 14:15). There enters a suffering fellow pilgrim. The first thing one consents to do is to welcome and listen. It is an act of love.

2. To Be a Companion

The willingness to enter into a helping relationship is essentially the willingness to be a companion — not a teacher, not a savior, but a companion. One agrees to go along. The word "companion" means one who breaks bread with another. People who break bread together share life. It might be nice to be able to do more for someone else — to be savior, wonder-worker, supplier of every need. The helper cannot promise so much, but one gift he or she can give, and that is to be a companion. I will go with you on your journey, take to heart all that concerns you, be there when you need me. This is companionship.

It is a limited role to be sure. But if it does nothing else it lifts the dread burden of loneliness from the shoulders of the other, and that makes all other burdens lighter. Camus' brief statement is an accurate utterance of the hope of one who opens his or her life to another.

Do not walk behind me. I may not lead.

Do not walk in front of me. I may not follow.

Just walk beside me, and be my friend.

The helper does not always solve the problem or take the pain away. But he or she is friend and resource, to explore with another, to watch another with concern, to listen and respond, to be available.

3. To Love

To listen attentively to another and to go with another in companionship are expressions of love. To do either without love is an empty gesture and bears no fruit. The helper loves the other. Now there is not a greater thing we can do for another human being than to love him or her. We touch here a truth just large enough to be easily overlooked. I am supposed to be a Christian helper, so I snap to attention. I put on a hat. I will be a sterling model of the Christian life, a shrewd analyst, an expert advisor. I will also develop a pep talk. These things have their place, but to put them first is to mistake the lesser for the greater. The most helpful thing one human being can do for another is to love him or her, and this is as valid for helping relationships as for any other kind.

Karl Menninger, after decades of work in psychotherapy, lays aside all learned talk both of psychic maladies and of therapeutic techniques, and utters one simple overarching truth: It is unlove that makes people unwell, and it is love and love alone that can make them well again. His contention is buttressed by more general studies and surveys, in which it has been shown that those therapists are most successful in bringing health back to their clients who are best able to convey love. Their theoretical framework may be Freudian, Jungian, Rogerian, Gestalt, Transactional Analysis, or anything else; the most telling factor is still the ability to communicate care, reverence, and hope to the troubled person. This explains in part why some psychotherapists seem to do so little for people even after months and years of appointments, and some complete amateurs are able to make a significant difference in a short time. In my own years of receiving spiritual direction from various directors, it is clear to me that those who helped me the most were not the eldest of them, the holiest, or the best schooled in counseling and spiritual direction; it was those who loved me the most. How did it work? They enabled me to believe in myself, to rejoice in my own being and gifts, to accept the mystery of my life in hope, and to make the most of it. Compared to this, analysis, advice, summaries of treatises, and exhortations to the heights come to very little.

Consider the effectiveness of Jesus, that great healer of the human spirit. He was not a trained therapist, nor even a trained priest or rabbi. He worked transformations in the lives of people because he loved them. He gave Magdalen a new lease on life because he loved her (Lk 7). He enabled Peter to become a fisher of human beings because he loved him in spite of himself (Lk 5). He got Zaccheus to come down from his tree and give half of his goods to the poor because he loved him (Lk 19). And he heals each of us in exactly the same way, accepting us in spite of our sinfulness, staying with us in spite of our waywardness, loving us in spite of everything that is wrong with us. This is what keeps the sun coming up in the morning. Love is creative and transformative power, coming into our lives always as the great surprise, filling our sails with a fresh breeze.

> And Jesus stopped and said, "Call him." And they called the
> blind man, saying to him, "Take heart; rise, he is calling you."
> And throwing off his mantle he sprang up and came to Jesus"
> (Mk 10:49-50).

How does one person love another? Love is partly a gift, partly a choice. One dimension of the experience of loving someone is gift: to me it is given deeply to understand and appreciate this person, and to care for him or her. Some individuals seem to have the capacity to love many people, and to love them easily. This is the first thing to look at when considering one's suitability for being a Christian helper. Am I the sort of person who genuinely likes people, who readily sees the good in them, who positively enjoys getting to know them? If so, then I have one of the basic gifts of the Christian helper.

Love is also partly a choice. It is the choice to respect another, to recognize his or her autonomy, to presume good will. It is the choice to welcome another warmly, and to provide an environment in which the other can feel safe. It is the choice to listen to another with attention and interest, to affirm and confirm all that one can, to share something of one's own experience, and to apologize when one offends. "Love is patient and kind," Paul says. "Love bears all things, believes all things, hopes all things, endures all things" (1 Cor 13:4-7). These are the choice aspects of love. The more one likes and feels enthusiasm for the person who comes, the easier it is to do these things. But even in the absence of such feelings, one can choose to do the deeds of love.

4. To Be Oneself

The helper is one who is willing to be him- or herself. Not a professional who hides behind a mask, but a fellow struggler of flesh and blood, with his or her own burdens, doubts, fears, weaknesses, temptations, guilt. To be oneself in a helping conversation might be to allow oneself to cry with one in deep sorrow, to express outrage as one listens to a person suffering injustice, to admit that one is just as baffled by the mystery of life and of God as one's puzzled friend. These are not studied or affected responses, given because calculated to be helpful, but the natural responses of heart and mind as one enters freely into the experience of another. To be oneself is the key, expressing puzzlement if puzzlement is felt, affirmation if affirmation is felt, disagreement if disagreement is felt — but all of these modestly, as having no more authority than that of one's personal reactions.

Presuming normal personal development, common sense, and a reasonable freedom from bias, simply to be oneself and to react naturally to what one hears is to be a reality principle in the life of the other. Everything that has been said so far about the role of the helper boils down to taking a genuine interest in and caring for the person. Now we are talking about what contributes to changing the person's perspective on reality. Each of us is limited in our perspectives on our own affairs. Each of us is a poor judge in our own case. To hear another agree and confirm, or simply understand and accept without condemning, or remind us of some obvious aspects of a situation we have overlooked in our pre-occupation with other aspects, or tell us rather obvious things about ourselves that we have forgotten — these are very helpful contributions to our self-understanding and our perceptions. We get down on ourselves, and another person speaks of our goodness and our gifts, which strike him or her as so much larger. We describe apparently insoluble dilemmas, and another person suggests possible courses of action we had never considered. We confess our hidden doubts and fears as problems uniquely our own, and another person makes us feel at home in the human race. We describe the world as constituted in a certain way, and another person says he or she sees it differently. We keep wrestling with and rearranging the superficial factors in a situation, and another person leads us to a deeper consideration and engagement of it. The helper in all these situations is doing nothing more complicated than being him- or herself, reacting naturally as a person's narrative unfolds, asking the questions, making the observations, sharing the feelings that occur. Thus the helper functions as a kind of reality principle, sometimes confirming, sometimes challenging the other to view things in a different light.

What It Is Not...

We can further clarify the helper's role if we look at some of the things it is not.

1. To Be Responsible for Another Person's Life

The helper does not take responsibility for the life of the other. To take that responsibility is first of all to assume a heavy burden, and a charge ultimately impossible to execute. Further it does a grave injustice to the person seeking help, since it keeps him or her in a position of dependency and immaturity. The temptation here is a subtle one, whose source may lie on either side of the relationship. The person seeking help may want to get rid of responsibility; the person offering help may positively relish dependents and authority. But this displacement is an unconscionable violation of mature personhood.

To the average person called upon to help another, as well as to the balanced person seeking help, the statement of this principle is an immense relief. Each, for good reasons, would avoid a relationship defined in dependency terms. But a relationship defined in mutually free and responsible terms is palatable. A qualification should be put in before we leave this point. This refusal to assume responsibility for another's life or to foster dependency does not mean we will let no one cry on our shoulder, come back a second time, ask for advice, or seek more companionship for a period than would be usual. There is a certain element of dependency in the very seeking of help. The point is that the ultimate objective will always be to give people's lives back to them, to help them make their own decisions and be responsible for them, to increase their sense of a healthy autonomy.

2. To Remove Problem and Pain

Another presumption that defeats helping relationships from the start is the helper's presumption that he or she is being asked to solve the problem or put an end to the suffering. This is usually impossible, and is rarely being asked for. But if the helper assumes that this is the assignment, there is bound to be anxiety, frustration, and a strong urge to flee all such situations. If, for example, someone is grieving over the loss of a spouse, there is no way the death can be undone or the pain taken away. If someone is dying of cancer, no conversation is going to avert death or abolish anguish. If a teenager is having trouble living in a home racked with marital conflict, he or she will most likely still be living there and trying to cope with the situation when the conversation is over. We do what we can to ameliorate problems and assuage sorrows. But there are a lot of human problems which cannot be solved, a lot of suffering that cannot be taken away. Usually when someone comes to us with a grief or a problem, he or she does not expect us to be able to change a situation very much if at all. It is something else they seek. Keeping that in mind makes the task a great deal easier to bear.

3. To Offer Greater Experience, Wisdom, and Holiness

Some misgivings besetting the helper stem from the presumption that one must be older, wiser, and holier than the person seeking help. All of these things might be considerable assets, but they are not strictly necessary. The great advantage the helper has is that he or she is distinct from the person seeking help, and so is not involved in the same way. A young spiritual director can often spot the self-deceptions of an older person, simply because they are quite obvious — except to the person suffering them. The director has self-deceptions too. We are all too close to ourselves, and vitally depend on the corrective supplied by an outsider's perspective. As with holiness, so with age and wisdom. One might have them in lesser measure than the one seeking help, and still be very useful just by reason of greater objectivity and ordinary insight.

The helper need not have had exactly the experience the other person is talking about. One can minister very effectively to the dying without having died oneself. One can be of assistance to the married without being married oneself. One can understand and help the homosexual without being gay oneself. Again here, having had the experience would usually be a great advantage — if one has the good sense to realize that the other's experience may not be precisely the same. But one need not have trod exactly the same winepress, because there are analogies in experience, and we can understand the other person's situation from experiences of our own which bear it some resemblance. One may not be a chronic depressive, and yet understand depression quite well from a personal brush with it. One may not be married, yet deal well with marital problems on the basis of having grown up in a family, having married friends, knowing the experience of friendship, and understanding something of male and female psychology. Thus, some priests have been fine marriage counselors. And a Roman Catholic sister who left her community told me that the person who understood her best was an older married man of a different race and a different faith. Empathy is the key, and some people have it in extraordinary measure.

There are times when we do *not* understand, and cannot enter the experience of another. These are not times to say, "I know just what you mean." They are rather times to say, "I've never had that experience myself. I wish I could understand it better." And sometimes we are asked questions to which the only truthful answer is: "That's something I guess I've never really thought about." Nothing is quite so refreshing as honesty, and it pays dividends in the long run, deepening the bond of trust. It gives the person the assurance that you will say what you really think, that you are not afraid, when the time is right, to say those three difficult words: "I don't know." Such an admission will usually not bring the conversation to a standstill. It may give it a push, inviting the other to elaborate and clarify what is not yet clear even to him- or herself. The helper will probably be brought to deeper insight too, or at least to further reflection.

4. To Make the Other a Different Person

It is salutary to face the limits of how much growth one may be able to occasion in the life of another. The other has a long history, a physical and psychic facticity, an ambience of impinging influences. It might be clear to us that what another person needs most is to fall in love. But it is difficult to make that happen. There are some marriages we would love to be able to save, and will not be able to. The alcoholic needs to stop drinking, the scrupulous person needs to put aside irrational anxieties, someone else needs to grow up. But we cannot make these things happen.

We may be directing someone's annual retreat, and, after listening to the person a few times, know clearly what grace he or she needs. But we cannot produce it, and may have miscalculated its opportuneness anyway. Human beings grow organically, and the operative factors in their growth are multiple, some environmental and some constitutional, all evasive of management. The helper is but one of those factors, and has only a modest function. One may be able to plant a seed in someone's mind that will bear fruit later. One may be able to help set up an occasion or situation which could foster the needed growth. But there are countless factors outside the helper's control, including the freedom of the person who comes. So the limits are sharply set. This can be very frustrating, but will be less so if one approaches helping relationships with realistic rather than unrealistic expectations. The butterfly cannot be made to emerge from the cocoon before it is time. And beagles are beagles. Here it is instructive to remember Paul's reflections on his work with other Christians.

> What then is Apollos? What is Paul? Servants through whom you believed, as the Lord assigned to each. I planted, Apollos watered, but God gave the growth. So neither the person who plants nor the person who waters is anything, but only God who gives the growth (1 Cor 3:5-7).

There is one important thing to remember when one is feeling inadequate to the challenge of a particular helping relationship, whether the root of the diffidence be apparently inferior qualifications, or an especially tough case. In most circumstances, the persons who came to you chose you. They did it for reasons which make sense at least to them. Just as they need help precisely because it is difficult for them to grasp their own situation, you might be suffering from the same lack of insight when you decide you cannot help them. One principle which may prove liberating in such situations, especially for those who tend to disparage themselves, is: If they are crazy enough to ask me, I'm crazy enough to say yes.

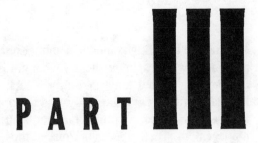

PRACTICAL APPROACHES FOR PASTORAL CARE

Overview

In the last section of this book, we hope to make some practical connections with the foundations laid out at the beginning. How do we intentionally create a pastoral care approach in our parishes, schools, communities, and families? How do we make pastoral care a priority component of all our ministry efforts? What are some of the resources available to us? What are the obstacles which confront us? How do we make pastoral care a collaborative effort?

Sharon Reed begins Part III by sketching the relationship between pastoral care and youth ministry. She looks at each of the components of youth ministry described in *A Vision of Youth Ministry* — word, worship, community, guidance and healing, justice and service, enablement, and advocacy — and suggests that pastoral care be woven into each of these dimensions of our youth outreach. Pastoral care is viewed as an attitude, opportunity, and action that faith communities take on behalf of youth people in general, rather than an approach used only in crisis situations. She encourages all of us to look for opportunities to be pastoral caregivers.

In Chapter 9 Joy Dryfoos identifies key ingredients of successful prevention programs drawn from her extensive research of over 100 programs.

In Chapter 10 Sharon Reed suggests a variety of strategies for effective pastoral care. Readers are encouraged to review the possibilities of mentoring, service programs, parent education, liturgy and ritual community networking and other creative ways of making pastoral care issues visible and viable to the faith community and the wider community.

In Chapter 11 we return to David Switzer for an essay on when and how to refer. Switzer looks at our limitations as primary and secondary caregivers and cautions against believing that we can handle anything and everything. He discusses situations that compel us to refer to other professionals, as well as some of the barriers to referral. Finally, Switzer challenges us to have the necessary resources at our fingertips, and to know how and where to refer for specific problems.

Reed then addresses the importance of an integrated approach to pastoral care in Chapter 12 by describing four fundamental approaches to planning, including a family perspective and community networking.

The book concludes with a listing of resources for pastoral care.

CHAPTER 8

YOUTH MINISTRY AND PASTORAL CARE

Sharon Reed

Over the years in youth ministry, one of the most valuable documents I ever read was *A Vision of Youth Ministry*. I found this vision to be quite expansive, forward-looking, idealistic yet grounded, and quite radical in its challenge. "The Church's youth ministry must be founded in the radical commitment to lay down one's life in service to the young people whose lives are touched" (*Vision* 4). Quite a serious pledge! "The vision of youth ministry must be understood and carried out in a manner that is grounded in scripture and gospel values and oriented to persons as fundamentally as Jesus' ministry was" (*Vision* 6). This meant a return to the style of Jesus — persons over institutions; relationships rather than programs! "Youth ministry works to foster the total personal and spiritual growth of each young person and to draw young people to responsible participation in the life, mission, and work of the faith community" (*Vision* 7). I was pretty amazed that the Church endorsed a document as radical as this one! How could we ever live up to its demands?

As I write this, many people would say that we've far exceeded its demands and many others would say that we still have a long way to go. Maybe the original concept was just too simple for our complicated lives. Maybe ministry grew too fast and many of the original priorities got squeezed out of the picture. Maybe we just got so sophisticated in our approach that we forgot the value of the original vision. We have definitely evolved, but the vision still remains our primary framework and there is still much to be done. We seem to have limited ourselves and now its time to break open that vision and allow it be seen through the lens of the '90s. There is still much we can be and that means *presence*:

> In some churches youth ministry is a struggle. Attendance is sporadic. The interests of young people are elsewhere. The activities are irrelevant... In other churches the youth program is highly successful in terms of numbers, activities and fun... Yet after three or four years of either type of youth program, small and struggling or big and eventful, a young person may not have heard the good news that God loves her, that she has an identity and purpose in life, that her sins are forgiven, that she is called into community, that she has support for her individuality and a place for corporate action and witness (Ng 49-50).

No, I'm not suggesting that we start over or fix something that isn't broken. However, I am suggesting a return to the principles of Jesus' ministry and the principles of the original vision statement. We must renew our commitment to young people in a clear and concrete way — pastoral care. Above all, pastoral care is a relationship. It is a process of attending to the needs of young people, their families, the parish, and wider community. Pastoral care is the original vision told through the Emmaus story. It involves healing, reconciling, sustaining, confronting, guiding and informing (Rowatt 22). It is growth toward wholeness and involves becoming, belonging, and transforming. For me, youth ministry and pastoral care are practically synonymous.

Pastoral care is simply not an option, but a key ingredient in what we are about as Church. "Youth ministry that calls forth a commitment will be a ministry in which adolescents resources are taxed and tested, in which their present capacities and skills are stretched to the limits, and in which the excitement and daring of being a Christian is experienced personally" (Dykstra 83). And it will be a ministry where adolescents are cared for, reached out to, empowered, invited, befriended, and transformed. "For us, as for the apostles, now is the time for action. The vision has been presented. There are many possibilities. It remains to be made a living reality" (*Vision* 26). Making the vision a reality has always been our call. How do we move it from the printed word and into our parish communities? How do we reach those young people who have never been part of our parish communities? Only a pastoral care approach can help young people feel visible and viable. We must commit ourselves to nurturing wholeness at each stage of the life journey, in the contexts that most influence young people — youth culture, society at large, their families, schools and local churches — and by presenting a prophetic witness and modeling an integrated approach to pastoral care in all aspects of youth ministry.

SUPPORTING ADOLESCENT TRANSITIONS

> The majority of young people emerge from adolescence healthy, hopeful, and able to meet the challenges of adult life. Half of America's 10-17 yr. olds are doing well and are at very low risk of experiencing problems related to their social behavior. They are progressing in school, they are not sexually active, they do not commit delinquent acts, and they do not use drugs or alcohol... Of great concern, however, are the one-quarter of American adolescents who engage in high-risk behaviors that endanger their own health and well-being and that of others as well. Special efforts must be made to reach these young people and provide them with both the means and motivation to avoid risky, dangerous and destructive activities that threaten their prospects for a satisfying adult life, their families, and their communities (*Beyond Rhetoric* 219-220).

What could possibly make the difference between these two experiences? For many young people it's the presence of special supportive adults — teachers, youth ministers, grandparents and parents, mentors, coaches, clergy — who provide encouragement and guidance when needed. Others had access to a broad array of community-based supports (Scouts, volunteer and service agencies, sports teams, counselors, bosses) who helped them discipline their time, identify their talents, and focus on someone else's need rather than their own. Still others had positive church experiences and were surrounded by adults and peers who promoted and modeled positive values and behaviors. Many cite families where parents and siblings spent time together. The challenge for youth ministry is to help foster reliable and caring attachments that encourage young people throughout their adolescent years. Carnegie Corporation President David Hamburg concluded that adolescents "need to find a place in a valued group, to engage in tasks the group considers valuable, to feel a sense of personal worth, and to have reliable, close relationships with others" (*Preparing for Life*).

One of the foundational principles of youth ministry has always been the importance of Catholic Christian role models who will affirm adolescent struggles, listen to their stories and questions, share their own faith journeys, and ask questions that encourage critical thinking and reflection. One of the foundational principles of pastoral care is the need for relationships built on mutual respect, availability, flexibility, and understanding. Both imply an ability to "be there" with an adolescent, to walk through the messes of our contemporary world, to challenge each other to grow, to learn from each other, and to witnesss to the God within and among us. Both call for the one-to-one model of ministry Jesus lived, yet remind us that true ministry duplicates itself. The challenge "involves the whole faith community speaking on behalf of these youth, and working for the resolution of the conflicts they face... young people need the example, fellowship, and acceptance of clergy, religious and lay adults to choose love, to choose community, and to choose faith" (*Vision* 11-12).

A pastoral care approach calls for a return to pastoring — an ongoing process of caring deeply and confronting honestly, of meeting people where they are and showing them the rich possibilities of human wholeness. It is the call for adolescents to believe in themselves because someone else already believes in them. After all, Jesus related to people in terms of what they could become as well as who they already were. Jesus' ability to see and affirm the potential within persons helped them develop the courage and strength to become caring followers and dynamic leaders. Certainly with that same attention young people are capable of doing the same! Pastoral care in the context of total youth ministry makes each young person feel special and important by offering intensive, individual attention.

Pastoral care also must touch the important people and institutions in the adolescent's life — parents, peers, parish, schools, community. All contexts of an adolescent's life must be included in the pastoral care network to avoid at-risk situations and promote healthy life choices. Pastoral care demands that we surround young people with the best adult support system possible. Are we willing to return to a ministry of compassionate presence as a standard requirement in our preferential option for the young? Are we willing to invest in the ministry of pastoring as a fundamental component of youth ministry? If not, how will we promote healthy adolescent development, as well as responsible participation in the life and mission of the Church? "Adults can and must help young people navigate this critical passage (between childhood and adulthood) by providing attention and guidance and by involving them in activities that offer hope and opportunity, prevent or remediate high-risk behaviors, bring the worlds of work and school closer together, and create opportunities for young people to contribute to the well-being of their communities" (*Beyond Rhetoric* 222). If young people have sufficient assets in their lives, particularly parents and other pastoral adults, even considerable challenges need not become insurmountable problems. Pastoral care and youth ministry go hand-in-hand. They derive from the same vision, point to the same priorities, arrive at the same conclusions, offer the same hope.

PASTORAL CARE AND THE YOUTH MINISTRY COMPONENTS

Clinebell describes pastoral care as the "utilization by persons in ministry of one-to-one or small group relationships to enable healing empowerment and growth to take place within individuals and their relationships" (26). At first glance, we might assume that guidance and healing is the only component of youth ministry that fosters such an outcome. In essence, the entire *Vision* statement is an endorsement and validation of the necessity for pastoral care, but particularly pastoral care as the bottom line in each of the seven components. In order to reenergize and revitalize our current approach to supporting positive adolescent development, we must integrate pastoral care into all that we are about as well as address the implications of a ministry rooted in pastoral care principles and perspectives.

Word (Evangelization and Catechesis)

"The fullest effectiveness of the ministry of the word requires sensitivity to many other aspects of youth ministry because youth need to experience the Christian message in terms of the realities most important in their daily lives: love, family, life values, justice, etc." (*Vision* 14). Are we really involved in teaching as Jesus did, in preaching the good news, in sharing the meaning and message of Jesus' ministry? Many of us are trapped in old models and are more loyal to the efficiency of the model, rather than the needs of the young people we serve. We are often obsessed by the quantity of information we have to impart, rather than the quality of the process. Pastoral care models would emphasize formation as well as information, youth input on both the topics and models, cate-chizing for justice and service, outreach to alienated young people through special offerings that respond to their issues, experiences of base Christian communities (RCIA, RENEW, peer ministry), challenging faith themes that promote the development of internal assets.

Christian education in the '90s needs to include more than just the learning of religious knowledge. Curriculum must be skills-based and highly experiential. Our classrooms must become laboratories where young people practice the how-to's of life as well as the how-to's of the Christian faith. We must equip them with skills which will empower them to be responsible adult followers of Christ (Rice 71). Retreats are a criti-cal component, but so are other opportunities which call for a networking of the wider community. Parents and family programs must be an integral priority. A new approach to planning and implementation will require greater interaction on many levels — parish, school, community resources — with an emphasis on the "total" development of the adoles-cent. If we want young people to commit to the Gospel message, we must be willing to commit to them as well.

Worship

"Worship builds and celebrates a relationship between God and peo-ple; it is a moment of personal and communal encounter with God" (*Vision* 16). Young people must be invited to participate in the sacramen-tal life of the Church. A pastoral care approach would highlight the role of the sacrament of Reconciliation in adolescent's personal healing process and in the healing of family, peer and other significant relation-ship. When we as Church are also responsible for rendering them powerless, we are responsible for healing that hurt. What better way to do this than through the sacraments? Young people need to be involved in anointing and healing services as well as other prayer experiences that involve the wider faith community. If our liturgical celebrations are expressions of our lived experience and if adolescents are in any way excluded from those celebrations, aren't we also denying the value of their experiences as reason to celebrate? The entire faith community must examine the way it worships together and what it says about not only its beliefs and values, but its relationship with each other and particularly what it says about its attitude and relationship particularly toward youth. "No person can be whole and remain isolated from meaningful related-ness" (Rowatt 24). Involvement in meaningful prayer and worship is crucial to further future self-investment in growth through outreach — an important goal of pastoral care.

Community

"In a community, youth have a mutual ministry to each other. They share themselves, their convictions, their faith... Building new paths of communication and providing opportunities for deeper levels of sharing are part of the ministry of creating intergenerational community" (*Vision* 16) In *A Different Drum*, Scott Peck claims that "community is currently rare." Many folks would second that comment in terms of today's Catholic Church. We need to be more intentional in our efforts to provide community-building opportunities. Community cannot be artificially created, but must be allowed to happen. Community provides continuity, and continuity allows for change. Pastoral care is about community, continuity, change and compassion. No single program can accomplish this, but only a comprehensive, integrated, ministry. We must re-focus on the role of the family. It is not enough to have a family perspective if it is not acted upon. Youth, singles, families of all shapes and sizes (with and without children), the elderly, all must be welcomed, attended to and responded to, challenged, and offered a "place" to be. The youth community is important, but there are so many ways for them to influence their families, friends, alienated youth, youth and community organizations, the political process. The four assets the Search Institutes sees as contributing to a reduction in risk-taking behaviors are primary examples of the powerful impact of positive community experiences: family support, positive school climate, involvement in structured extracurricular activities in community and school, and involvement in a church or synagogue. Can youth ministry possibly aim for less?

Guidance and Healing

"Youth ministry responds to the profound needs of modern youth for spiritual and personal counseling, for vocational guidance, and for the reconciliation that heals the wounds of alienation... Good communication and cooperation among the many agencies established to serve youth are a vital aspect of an effective ministry of guidance" (*Vision* 17). If there is any component where youth ministry and pastoral care are obviously and intimately linked, it is this one. Ironically, it may also be the component that has received the least attention since the *Vision* statement was published. I think we're very uncomfortable with the words "guidance" and "healing," yet both were at the heart of Jesus' mission and ministry. Maybe it's the feeling that as youth ministers we must be adept and expert at each of these components and this makes us feel rather inadequate. A classic example of good pastoral care is to be in touch with our own limitations and surround young people with adults who are best able to meet a given need. Are there spiritual directors available for those adolescents who might want to pursue their spiritual journey on a one-to-one basis? Who are the counselors in the community best equipped to deal with adolescent and family issues from a sound value stance? What kind of direct aid is your parish community willing or able to provide to families in crisis? What direct aid is available to youth-at-risk (resources, referrals, skill development programs, peer ministry, etc.)? What's already happening in the community at large that you can tap into? What support groups are already in existence? Do any community youth services ever use parish facilities? The possibilities for pastoral care here are endless. Someone must begin to take notice!

Justice and Service

"As a natural outflowing of the community experience of faith service and action on behalf of justice should be constitutive dimensions of the Church's youth ministry" (*Vision* 18). Pastoral care is not simply a private, personal agenda, or a me-me, me-God approach. It continually calls us to consider the ways in which racism, militarism, sexism, economic and political exploitation cripple our search for wholeness on a much wider scale. "To correct this myopia, the pastoral care of groups and institutions must be seen as the other side of personal and relational healing and growth work... There can be no full or long-term wholeness for individuals and families in a broken world, a world that destroys wholeness by its systems of injustice, violence, poverty and exploitation" (Clinebell 33). Youth ministry through pastoral care strives to promote the dignity of all persons through responsible Christian action. Poverty, violence, unemployment and sexism are rapidly infiltrating the world of the adolescent. Youth must be challenged not to remain self-conscious, but other-conscious. Pro-active behavior on behalf of others has continually been noted as an asset to healthy development. In addition, the Church's stance is equally important — an institutional model of Christian values in action. Pastoral care means responding to those young people who are victims themselves, raising the consciousness of all young people to local concerns and global needs, and empowering them to work for change. Youth ministry thus promotes capable, confident, compassionate, caring young people — a goal shared again with pastoral care.

Enablement/Leadership Development

"Young people should be welcomed as co-workers in youth ministry, and programs which develop their leadership talents should have a central place" (*Vision* 18). Training is an essential instrument for renewal in our Church. It can assist our potential for authenticity and creativity. Young people need the opportunity not only to identify their gifts but also to have them nurtured and enhanced. They also need to address the skills they are lacking and be trained in areas critical to future roles. "Youth need to learn how to make decisions, how to communicate with others, how to solve problems, how to think critically, how to plan, how to get things done. They need to learn responsibility and self-control. Human beings are not born with these skills" (Rice 71).

Adults need quality formation programs as well if ministry to youth is really to be taken seriously. We cannot expect quality care for our young people unless quality care is provided for the adults who minister to and with them. Pastoral care suggests training programs based on solid theological underpinnings, solid ministerial skills, spiritual formation, and understanding of adolescent issues and development. Pastoral care of youth ministers promotes reasonable job descriptions, just salaries and benefits, opportunities for spiritual direction and spiritual enrichment, and attention to the family and personal needs they bring with them. A holistic approach to training and evaluation and support is imperative! The quality of presence an adult brings to youth ministry depends in large part on the quality of presence in their own lives and in their faith community!

Advocacy

"An advocate for youth shows dedication by interpreting and speaking for youth before the Church and secular community. Advocacy gets down to the everyday practicality of being a buffer, an intermediary, a broker" (*Vision* 21). Once again we're back to the need for adult presence — mentors, supporters, those who will keep young people visible in today's Church, those who will lobby for youth services, who will value the unique contribution and wisdom of youth as persons, not commodities, or consumers. Pastoral care through advocacy is a means to "allow the direction of another's growth to guide what I do, to help determine how I am to respond and what is relevant to such response. I appreciate the other as independent in his/her own right with needs that are to be respected" (Mayeroff 5). Jesus acted as an advocate for many on the fringes of society — women, children, sinners, the poor, the outcast, the different. We are obliged to continue that response in every aspect of youth ministry. We are in a covenant relationship with these young people. We must remind bishops, clergy, parents, and the wider community of that enormous responsibility. Our youth programs must be rooted in a belief that young people are called by their baptism to full, conscious, and active involvement in the life and mission of the Church. Only then will we be transformed by their wisdom and grace. Youth ministry has too long been silenced — a prophetic voice is essential.

THE CHALLENGE OF PASTORAL CARE

We are deeply entrenched, most of us, in the ministries and institutions of the past... It is not enough for us to have institutions that are viable. The institutions we have must also be truly prophetic... It is not the continuation of what we have done well in the past that must be our concentration; it is the cry of the present to which we must attend if we are to be authentic. It is not witness by withdrawal from the great questions of life that will determine our value; it is being "in the world but not of it"... We will not be forgiven our indifference (Chittister 152).

Joan Chittister used these words to sum up the challenges facing her own Benedictine community. They can equally be applied to the major challenges facing the pastoral care of youth. We will not be forgiven our indifference to young people, to their families, and the healthy development of both. That is why pastoral care can no longer be viewed as an option, an alternative to fall back on when other strategies seem to fail. Our challenge is to create more connections for young people through family and community support programs, and to improve the number and quality of programs already in existence. We cannot remain in our comfortable oasis of a weekly youth group, but must emphasize prevention and intervention when necessary. Even though much good has been done, there is still much that demands our attention. We need "an overall pastoral approach" with a focus on "the truth about Jesus Christ, the truth about the Church's mission, and the truth about the human being" (*Puebla and Beyond* 269).

Pastoral care is an integral part of the faith community's responsibility to its young. There is a growing need for collaboration and cooperation, not competition, among other ministries as well as other youth serving agencies. Young people need the freedom to move in and out of new relationships, test different groups, choose from a variety of options, and have input into the decision-making process. Adaptability and availability are key issues. Healthy adolescent growth and development are too important to put on the back burner.

A recommitment to *A Vision of Youth Ministry* means a recommitment to pastoral care. Although many teenagers navigate through adolescence quite successfully, many do not. More than 50% of today's teenagers are sexually active. Approximately 1.3 million teenagers have a serious drinking problem. Five thousand teenagers commit suicide each year and fifty to one hundred make an unsuccessful attempt for each successful one. Crime rates among juveniles have increased among juveniles and young people are often the victims of violence. Over one million children run away from home each year (Elkind 7-8). Even those who demonstrate remarkable resiliency during this period seem to lack a clearly defined value system, the time and space to form a distinct sense of self, and a stress-free atmosphere in which to pursue their own issues. Young people need to not only deepen their relationship with God, but to renew their intimate relationships (particularly within the family) and grow in relationship to the significant institutions of their world. Holistic pastoral care enables adolescents to balance growth in all these areas. They need to be liberated, empowered, and nurtured if they are to truly experience the gospel as good news and share it with others. Therefore, we must commit ourselves to a specific pastoral care agenda for all our youth ministry efforts. I would like to propose five elements of this pastoral care agenda:

1. Be Proactive. "The proactive choice is to change from the inside-out: to *be* different, and by being different to effect positive change in what's out there" (Covey 89). As Church, we must change ourselves before we can effect change. We have to stop empowering outside conditions to control our attitudes and direction.

2. Begin to Organize Around Pastoral Care as a Priority. We must be intentional about integrating pastoral care approaches and programs into our comprehensive youth ministry. We must reexamine the quality of our presence to and with young people and make needed changes. We must plan for effectiveness and not merely efficiency.

3. Create a Balanced Focus Between Doing and Increasing Our Ability to Do. Adults need on-going training to deal with pastoral care issues. More and more time and energy must be devoted to expand the available pool of adults to serve as mentors and role models, trainers, supporters, and professional youth minsters. Adults who are willing to identify, research, and investigate available community resources will be in demand. Youth ministry and pastoral care will demand a team effort, a balance of being and doing competently.

4. Make Parents and Families a Primary Target. We have barely scratched the surface in our pastoral care of families. Much more needs to be done than simply to be aware of family time when scheduling programs. What are the inherent needs of families with adolescents — parent support groups, prayer groups, education on adolescent development, family activities and liturgies, counseling services and resources, latchkey programs? Parents are at a loss for answers. Certainly the Church has a role in helping them deal with the questions. What about single-parent families and their distinct needs? How do we respond to cultural diversity within our parishes? Family ministry and youth ministry need to join forces to deal with these complex issues.

5. Create a Spillover Effect. The entire faith community cannot help but be affected when we're dealing with issues that affect our personal, spiritual, physical, emotional, and mental health. But everyone needs to be brought on board. We need to abandon our fragmented, disconnected ministry approaches, where the right hand has no idea what the left is doing. Again, we must return to ownership of the vision. We must communicate with each other and take more responsibility for pastoral leadership. We must be welcoming, hospitable, *caring* communities. Someone must take the initiative of *voicing* the concern. The possibilities are endless.

> The natural human spirit is irrepressibly radical; it wants the unattainable, years for the impractical, is willing to risk the improper. But as we conform ourselves to the practicalities and proprieties of efficiency, we restrict the space between desire and control; we confine our intention to an ever-decreasing range of possibilities. The choices we make — and therefore the way we feel about ourselves — are determined less by what we long for and more by what is controllable and acceptable to the world around us. After enough of this, we lose our passion. We forget who we are. It is imperative, not just for our individual spiritual growth but for the hope of the world, that we begin to reverse this process (May 47).

Pastoral care is all about restoring the passion and reminding us who we are. Can we honestly afford to risk losing the passion and identity of our young people or ourselves? I think not!

Works Cited

Beyond Rhetoric: A New American Agenda for Children and Families. National Commission on Children, 1991.

Chittister, Joan. *Woman Strength: Modern Church, Modern Women.* Kansas City, MO: Sheed and Ward, 1990.

Clinebell, Howard. *Basic Types of Pastoral Care and Counseling.* Nashville: Abingdon Press, 1984.

Covey, Stephen. *The 7 Habits of Highly Effective People.* New York: Simon and Schuster, 1989.

Dykstra, Craig. "Agenda for Youth Ministry: Problems, Questions, and Strategies." *Readings and Resources in Youth Ministry* (Warren, Ed.) Winona, MN: St. Mary's Press, 1987.

Elkind, David. *All Grown Up and No Place to Go.* New York: Addison-Wesley Pub., 1984.

Hamburg, David. *Preparing for Life: The Critical Transition of Adolescence.* New York: Carnegie Corporation of New York, 1986.

May, Gerald. *The Awakened Heart.* New York: Harper Collins Pub., 1991.

Mayeroff, Milton. *On Caring.* New York: Harper and Row, 1971.

Ng, David. *Youth in the Community of Disciples.* Valley Forge, PA: Judson Press, 1984.

Rice, Wayne. "An Agenda for Youth Ministry in the 90's." *Youthworker*, spring, 1990.

Rowatt, G. Wade. *Pastoral Care with Adolescents in Crisis.* Louisville: John Knox Press, 1989.

A Vision of Youth Ministry. Washington, DC: USCC, 1976.

CHAPTER 9

COMMON COMPONENTS OF SUCCESSFUL PREVENTION PROGRAMS

Joy G. Dryfoos

(Editor's Note: The following common components of successful prevention programs is based on the analysis of 100 prevention programs by Joy Dryfoos. She extracted from each of the program description the specific items that characterized the intervention. For some programs, information about components was compiled from monographs or site visits and was rich in detail. For other programs, information was compiled from the literature, organization reports, or responses to telephone queries. What follows is an impressionistic overview of available data by Dryfoos. Many diverse program components were identified in the program

descriptions that fell into categories such as timing, staffing, participants, program operations, personal support, specific skills, and incentives. Each program was characterized by four to six items. Those components that were most prevalent in each of the four different fields conclusively surfaced to the top and are described in the following discussion as the common components of successful programs. She concludes that the most significant finding from this exercise was the remarkable co-occurrence of specific components in each of the diverse fields of prevention.)

LESSONS FROM THE MODELS

Some 11 common program components emerged from an analysis of the reported practices in successful intervention programs. Of these, the first two appeared to have the widest application: *the importance of providing individual attention to high-risk children and the necessity for developing broad communitywide interventions.* These items represent two points at either end of a spectrum that extends from individual one-on-one support to institutional changes in the community. This finding supports the view that the needs of high-risk children must be met at the personal level within the context of broader changes in the social environment.

1. Intensive Individualized Attention

In successful programs, high-risk children are attached to a responsible adult who pays attention to that child's specific needs. This theme was operationalized in each of the fields in several different kinds of programs. In substance abuse prevention, a student assistance counselor was available full-time for individual counseling and referral for treatment. In delinquency prevention, a family worker from the alternative diversion project gave "intensive care" to a predelinquent and the family to assist them to make the necessary changes in their live to avoid repeat delinquent acts. In pregnancy prevention, a full-time social worker placed in the school system was available for individual counseling and referral. In school remediation, a prevention specialist worked with very high-risk children and their families to improve school attendance.

Various techniques were used, including individual counseling and small group meetings, individual tutoring and mentoring, and case management. Both professionals (psychologists, social workers, counselors, teachers) and nonprofessionals (community aides, volunteers) were utilized in these efforts. Personal counseling and support were offered in preschool settings, school classrooms, "time-out" rooms, school-based clinics, alternative schools, afterschool programs, community agencies, and through home visits and outreach.

2. Community-wide Multiagency Collaborative Approaches

The operating hypotheses of these community-wide programs is that, to change the behavior of young people, a number of different kinds of programs and services have to be in place. This theme was exemplified in the substance abuse prevention field by a community-wide health promotion campaign that used local media and community education in conjunction with the implementation of substance abuse prevention curricula in the local school. In the delinquency prevention field, the neighborhood development program involved local residents in neighborhood councils, working with the schools, police, courts, gang leaders, and the media. A successful model in pregnancy prevention concentrated on community education through media and a speakers' bureau, training of parents, clergy, and other community leaders, and development and implementation of a comprehensive sex and family life education program in the schools. The problem of dropping out of school was addressed by an all-out community effort involving the schools with local businesses, local government agencies, and universities in planning, teacher training, and student training and job placement.

The multicomponent methodology builds on significant successes among community programs for heart disease prevention. [1] Experience with collaborative programs appears to be growing in all fields of prevention. Partners in the models included schools, community health and social agencies, businesses, media, church groups, universities, police and courts, and youth groups. The composition of the coalition depended on the particular "crisis" to which the community was responding (e.g., drugs, dropout rates, teen pregnancy, crime, suicide, etc.) Typically, multiagency efforts have representative advisory councils and use volunteers from the community for various tasks (e.g., planning, community information, grants), as well as for personal mentoring. Cooperation with local media is generally used for gaining access to channels through which education and consciousness-raising efforts can be brought to the community. Local businesses offer mentors, equipment, and incentives, act as role models for career education, and help with job training and placement.

3. Early Identification and Intervention

Reaching children and their families in the early stage of the development of problem behaviors demonstrated both short- and long-term benefits. One well-documented preschool program (Perry Preschool) served as a model for delinquency, pregnancy, and substance abuse prevention, as well as for school achievement. (In this case, careful longitudinal tracking of a very small sample produced significant results.) Other successful programs were directed toward preschoolers living in disadvantaged neighborhoods or elementary school students who were acting out in early grades or falling behind in achievement. Early needs assessments and computerized systems for tracking high-risk students over time are utilized in several programs.

4. Locus in Schools

Many of the successful prevention models are physically located in schools. We would expect that most school remediation and much of the substance abuse prevention would take place on school sites. However, it is of great significance that so many of the delinquency prevention and pregnancy prevention interventions were also located in schools. Of course, the goals of the interventions are interrelated, with the acquisition of basic skills as the bottom line for most high-risk children. The idea that a healthy, safe school climate and effective school organization contribute to prevention of negative behavior extends beyond the education field to the other prevention fields as well. Programs in which the principal is considered one of the key elements of success may be found across the various fields — for example, in school reorganization, on school teams for delinquency and substance abuse prevention, as facilitator for school-based clinics, and as liaison with student assistance counselors. Alternative schools and schools within schools have demonstrated improved behavioral as well as educational outcomes for high-risk youth.

5. Administration of School Programs by Agencies Outside of Schools

In each of the fields, agencies and organizations outside of the schools carried the major responsibility for exemplary programs that were implemented within the schools. Four types of arrangements were exemplified among the models: (1) the program was designed by a university-based researcher (e.g., James Comer at Yale or Cheryl Perry at Minnesota) who obtained a grant to implement the program and conducted evaluation research in the school or community agency; (2) the model was designed by a nonprofit youth services and research organization (e.g., Public/Private Ventures or the Academy for Educational Development) and implemented in multiple demonstration projects in schools or communities with support from foundations or government agencies; (3) a model was initiated by a foundation (e.g., Robert Wood Johnson, Annie E. Casey) or a government agency (e.g., Office of Substance Abuse Prevention, New Jersey Department of Human Services) which issued a request for proposals calling for comprehensive collaborative programs in schools; (4) a program was developed by a local health or youth service agency in collaboration with a school (Adolescent Resources Corporation in Kansas City) and obtained funds from a state health agency (Missouri Health Department) and foundations. In these types of interventions, project staff may work for the outside agency or be responsible for training and supervising on-site staff. Curriculum materials are usually created by program developers who also are available to provide technical assistance. In all cases, research is conducted by the outside agency. Schools typically provide space, maintenance, and coordination between outside agency staff and school personnel.

6. Location of Programs Outside of Schools

Not every successful program is located within a school. The staff of certain program models believe they are more effective because they are community rather than school based. Young people who are "turned off" by the school system were reported to have participated in programs in community and church centers, businesses, and a large array of youth service programs. Community-based youth-serving agencies appear to have greater latitude in offering controversial services, such as family planning, and can facilitate weekend and summer programs. Youth programs located outside of schools were able to offer a wide range of services; for example, many community centers had extensive arts programs with theater groups and painting classes. Others were geared up to serve the most high-risk populations, such as homeless and runaway youth, often providing overnight shelter. [2]

7. Arrangement for Training

Many of the successful programs employ special kinds of staff, professional or nonprofessional, who require training to implement a program. Often they are called on to use a certain protocol (behavioral therapy) or a new curriculum (Life Skills training). School reorganization entails complex concepts such as school-based management, team teaching, and cooperative learning. These approaches require extensive in-service training and ongoing supervision. A number of the model programs have established school teams, generally made up of the support personnel (social worker, psychologist, counselor), the school principal, in some instances parents, and occasionally students. These teams also require training and orientation to carry out the mandates of the intervention. Several model programs employ full-time staff to coordinate teams, curriculum development, treatment services, and referrals, as well as to expedite research protocols.

8. Social Skills Training

A number of variants of personal and social skills training have emerged in this review (and more exist than have been discussed). The approach generally involves teaching youngsters about their own risky behavior, giving them the skills to cope with and, if necessary, resist the influences of their peers in social situations, and by helping them to make healthy decisions about their futures. Techniques such as role-playing, rehearsal, peer instruction, and media analysis are typically employed. While much of the impetus for these curricula emerged from successes in smoking prevention, curricula currently in use are designed to prevent a range of behaviors with negative consequences. Examples have been given that resulted in delaying initiation of alcohol and marijuana use, delaying initiation of sexual intercourse, improving use of contraception, and improving behavior in school. Few of the social skills programs have demonstrated positive effects with high-risk children. What the research has documented is significant changes among participants that are maintained over a few years, especially if they are exposed to booster (repeat) sessions in subsequent years of school.

9. Engagement of Peers in Interventions

Program designers in every field are aware of the importance of peer influences on adolescent behavior. Research on the efficacy of using peers in prevention interventions has produced mixed results. However, several successful models emerged from this review. The most successful approaches use older peers to influence or help younger peers, either as classroom instructors (in social skills training) or as tutors and mentors. In some programs the peer tutors are paid. The training and supervision of the students are important aspects of this component.

Students selected to act as peer mentors gain the most from the experience, probably because of the intensive individual attention and enrichment they receive.

10. Involvement of Parents

While programs report less success in involving parents than they would like, a number of models across the various fields have demonstrated that programs directed toward parents can be successful. Two approaches have shown documented results: home visits that provide parent education and support, and employment of parents as classroom aides. Outreach to the homes of high-risk families has proven effective for adolescents as well as for preschool and other age children. Parents have also been recruited as members of school teams and advisory committees. It appears that the more defined the expected role for parents, the more likely that participation will occur. Invitations to attend meetings and workshops have failed to recruit the parents of high-risk children. Parent-training programs have been shown to be effective with selective groups.

11. Link to the World of Work

Programs in a variety of fields use innovative approaches to introduce career planning, expose youngsters to work experiences, and prepare them to enter the labor force. Successful models offered various components: combining life-planning curricula with school remediation and summer job placement; creating opportunities for volunteer community service; and paying high-risk youth to become tutors for younger children. These components were most often combined with group counseling and seminars to help students interpret and integrate the experience.

RECOMMENDATIONS FROM THE EXPERTS

In general, the experts' opinions confirm the lessons learned from the models. This is not unexpected when one considers that a number of the experts are responsible for the theoretical constructs that shape the models. There is an overlap between those who conduct the research and create the literature and those who are on the panels of experts that make recommendations to commissions and task forces. What is more important here than chicken-and-egg questions (Does the theory drive the practice or does the practice shape the theory?) is the significant agreement among the four diverse fields about concepts. Again, there is a striking consensus among experts from widely divergent disciplines about what needs to be done to help high-risk children.

Common Concepts Among Experts

Six major points surfaced in each of the problem areas, demonstrating the high level of agreement about solutions among the experts from different fields. These theoretical concepts strongly support the lessons learned from successful programs.

1. There Is No One Solution to This Problem

There is no single program component (no "magic bullet") that by itself can alter the outcomes for all children at high risk for delinquency, substance abuse, teen pregnancy, and school failure.

2. High-risk Behaviors Are Interrelated

Prevention programs should have broader, more holistic goals. Interventions should be directed at risk factors rather than at categorical problem behaviors.

3. A Package of Services Is Required Within Each Community

The package must contain multiple components that respond to the particular needs in that community. Community-wide planning is a requisite for bringing all the institutions together to determine what must be done.

4. Interventions Should Be Aimed at Changing Institutions Rather Than at Changing Individuals

The main thrust of prevention should be in the schools because low achievement is a major risk factor for each of the problems. The acquisition of basic skills is fundamental. Furthermore, schools should be the locus for nonacademic interventions that deal with health, welfare, and support because that's where the children are located, at least in their earlier years.

5. The Timing of Interventions Is Critical

Preschool and middle school periods are significant transition points in a child's life when major setbacks can occur. The middle school years have received the least attention in the past. Most interventions start too late to have any effect.

6. Continuity of Effort Must Be Maintained

"One shots" do not have any effect. Follow-up services, staff supervision, and booster curricula are necessary to insure that whatever changes take place are maintained.

End Notes

[1] For a review of the three major comprehensive communitywide prevention programs, see C. Johnson and J. Solis, "Comprehensive Community Programs for Drug Abuse: Implications of the Community Heart Disease Prevention Programs for Future Research." In T. Glynn, C. Leukefeld, and J. Ludford, Eds., *Preventing Adolescent Drug Abuse: Intervention Strategies* (National Institute on Drug Abuse, USDHHS, NIDA Research Monograph, 47, 1985): 76-114.

[2] A number of very impressive community programs were not included in the program models because they have never been evaluated or they didn't fit into any specific categorical notch. For example, *El Puente* (a Holistic Center for Growth and Development in Brooklyn, NY) serves large numbers of Hispanic youth and their families with health services, classes in karate and aerobics, a wide range of arts classes, counseling, and legal and social services; *Project Spirit* is a family-oriented church-based program operated by the National Congress of Black Churches in 15 churches in three cities. The project offers after-school tutorials, cultural enrichment, parent education, and a pastoral counseling education component. These programs, and many others, are described in the publications of the Adolescent Pregnancy Prevention Clearinghouse of the Children's Defense Fund.

CHAPTER 10

STRATEGIES FOR EFFECTIVE PASTORAL CARE

Sharon Reed

In their book *Raising Self-Reliant Children in a Self-Indulgent World*, H. Stephen Glenn and Jane Nelson propose strategies to "inoculate our children against developing the characteristics of high-risk individuals" (234-235). If there were such a "vaccine," I'm sure we would want to make it available to every parent and youth worker. Until such foolproof prevention exists, we will have to utilize the best proven strategies that we have for effective pastoral care and remember the wisdom Glenn and Nelson share near the end of their book:

> All we will ever get on this planet is one step at a time. All we'll ever be allowed to see is that first step, and it will be different for each of us because our eyes are all at different heights above the ground. The amount of confidence differs. Our legs are of different lengths. No one can take anyone else's first step... Choose just one thing you would like to work on. Make it something that

seems simple to you, perhaps eliminating a single barrier. Take that first step and you will see the next emerging from the dark. (Unfortunately), many people spend their whole life standing in the doorway (Glenn and Nelson 234).

We have all spent our share of time standing in the doorway, hoping for that flash of insight that would provide the perfect solution. As a Church, have we been standing around waiting too long? Young people in our country are refusing to be invisible. They are demanding our time and attention, as well as our prophetic action. It is our responsibility to "face the nature and scope of these problems and their growing severity and to take responsibility in the shared cooperative way throughout society" (Hamburg 13).

Youth ministers have always been aware of the fragile nature of the adolescent's world, yet there was so much that needed immediate attention that planning ahead was virtually impossible. Now what were once long range issues have become critical and urgent calls for action today — too close and too loud to ignore. We must use a variety of strategies to promote and sustain the growth (if not merely the survival) of the adolescents to whom we minister. The destination is clear. The journey is difficult. The directions are many.

This book proposes a broad understanding of pastoral care which includes three elements: *promotion* and *prevention* — strategies for promoting healthy adolescent development, *caring for youth in crisis* — strategies for responding through direct assistance to youth in need, and *advocacy* — strategies for challenging systems. As we saw in Chapter 8, pastoral care cannot be confined to the "guidance and healing" component of youth ministry, nor to one-on-one encounters with young people. Therefore, pastoral care cannot remain one person's responsibility — at the parish, community or regional levels. Task forces and teams of youth advocates are designing strategies to provide coping skills, multi-level support systems, parental involvement, and agendas for the present as well as the future.

This chapter will propose a variety of potential and proven strategies that can be employed to provide *preventive* pastoral care for adolescents and their families. Effective strategies need to be intense, comprehensive, and flexible. Together with the strategies for promoting healthy adolescent development in Chapter 2, the following strategies offer specific and adaptable approaches for pastoral care in local settings.

LIFE SKILLS TRAINING

"Clearly, today's adolescents need life skills training — the formal teaching of requisite skills for surviving, living with others and succeeding in a complex society" (Hamburg 241). Beatrix Hamburg, who chaired the Carnegie Council on Adolescent Development's Working Group on Life Skills Training, suggests that we must identify "core skills" that seem to have a universal bearing on different social groups and different communities. "Two prime candidates for such focus are *social skills* (non-violent conflict resolution, friendship formation, peer resistance, assertiveness, and renegotiation of relationships with adults) and *decision-making*" (Hamburg iv). Both of these have lifelong consequences and have a powerful impact on those with whom adolescents interact. We are operating in a world where guidelines for behavior are not very clear to adolescents or their parents. Many young people (due to divorce and remarriage) spend time in single parent or stepfamilies where guidelines are more difficult to enforce or several sets of guidelines are proposed, often in opposition to each other. The media is only to quick to jump in with another set of values and a variety of alternative messages and choices. So far, little has been done with media literacy and critical viewing skills, which makes life skills training more and more important if young people are to be significant contributors in designing their future.

H. Stephen Glenn and Jane Nelson speak of life skills in terms of the *significant seven*:

1. strong perceptions of personal capabilities ("I am capable");

2. strong perceptions of significance in primary relationships ("I contribute in meaningful ways");

3. strong perceptions of personal power ("I can influence what happens to me");

4. strong intrapersonal skills (understand emotions, develop self-discipline and self-control, and learn from experience);

5. strong interpersonal skills (develop friendships through communication, cooperation, negotiation, sharing, listening);

6. strong systemic skills (responsibility, adaptability, flexibility, integrity);

7. strong judgmental skills (evaluate situations according to appropriate values) (Glenn and Nelson 48-50).

Youth ministry has often concentrated on relationship skills, listening and communication skills, and leadership skills but never in a sustained, comprehensive program aimed at preventing problem behaviors and promoting healthy coping skills. Once the skills are learned, young people also need to be assisted in making applications to their everyday experience. These generic skills taught and learned in combination seem to prove more effective than single-issue prevention programs aimed at decreasing teenage pregnancy, drug and alcohol use, violence, etc. They challenge us to identify multiple skills which provide a solid foundation for dealing with a wide variety of life issues. In the best-selling book, *The 7 Habits of Highly Effective People*, these are defined as the "intersection of knowledge, skills, and desire" (Covey 47). I think this is what the crux is in our schools, youth programs and communities — we have effectively provided the knowledge and are just now beginning to translate that into "how" (the skill), while not yet tapping into the "want to do" (desire). "Even if I do know that in order to interact effectively with others I really need to listen to them, I may not have the skill... But knowing I *need* to listen and knowing *how* to listen is not enough. Unless I have the desire it won't be a habit in my life" (Covey 47). The skill is a critical link that hooks together knowledge and desire. Thus, young people need to apply and practice the skills they learn or old patterns of self-defeating behavior will never change and adolescents will remain paralyzed and powerless.

This situation is magnified in young people who are already considered to be at-risk — those who lack dependable family, school, and community environments and are at high-risk of engaging in multiple problem behaviors. Winthrop Adkins cites several different patterns necessary in life skills programs aimed at "disadvantaged" youth.

1. Structured, problem focused sessions with prepared materials/exercises.

2. Need to build general and specific knowledge base — group members often cannot act as resources for each other.

3. Common basis for interaction must be established — need to learn to talk each other's language.

4. Peer influence is high — can be used for peer teaching/cooperative learning.

5. Ability to handle stress is poor (Hamburg 243).

There are many model life skills programs being targeted toward specific issues throughout the country. Regardless of the make-up of the young people in your faith community, life skills training is one area where we cannot continue to stand in the doorway. Parishes and schools need to identify skills that are lacking and work with other community agencies. Some life skills need to be woven into religious education/youth ministry activities. Now is the time to commit personnel and resources.

Networks and Social Supports

It is evident that young people today turn more frequently to peers and other influences for support, values, and behavioral cues. Most adolescents grow up in dual career families with little access to relatives or extended family. Neighborhoods change rapidly because of the changing employment and economic situation. Many neighborhood schools are a thing of the past. Gangs are on the rise and young people are vulnerable to violent crimes we never experienced growing up.

> High risk youth in impoverished communities urgently need social support networks. These can be created in a wide-range of existing settings, such as school sports, school-based health clinics, community organizations, mentoring programs, home-visiting programs, and *church-related youth activities*. To be successful, the support networks must have dependable infrastructure and foster enduring relationships with adults as well as peers (Hamburg 253).

In addition to studying the crucial need for support systems for high-risk youth, the Carnegie Working Group identified the ingredients of effective support programs.

1. They respond to more than one serious problem or risk factor.

2. They take developmental information into account.

3. They create incentives that adolescents are likely to perceive as relevant to their own lives.

4. They open up social roles that are respected and provide adolescents opportunities to learn new skills.

5. They have relatively clear expectations and provide a predictable environment.

6. They foster active participation.

7. They may foster relationships among several support elements/systems.

8. They provide considerable continuity.

9. They build upon organizational readiness (Hamburg 254-256).

How many of these ingredients are readily apparent in your youth ministry? Just the fact that youth ministry exists proves the need for increasing the availability of social, spiritual, intellectual, and emotional support networks. How much more powerful our youth ministry efforts would be if we were closely connected to families, schools, and other community agencies who hold similar values and hopes for the future of our children. What can we be doing to raise the awareness of existing networks and to increase our connectedness? For one thing, we need to be much more aware of the services offered within our local, diocesan, and state communities and how to plug adolescents into these services. We need to be much more consultative and collaborative in working with those groups who influence our young people — including other churches, high schools, social service agencies, YMCA/YWCA, Young Life, sports teams, etc. Many times we seem to compete for the same resources rather than cooperatively utilize them. We also need to join forces with libraries, hospitals, social-service agencies, and businesses to lobby for change. As voters and taxpayers, we must support value-based issues that impact families and their children. What support groups operate that could meet in parish facilities? Young people risk being isolated unless we, as youth ministers, can help foster radical relatedness.

COMMUNITY INVOLVEMENT AND SERVICE

Certainly one way of solidifying the positive impact of social networks is to engage adolescents actively in creating their own personal impact. It has been noted that self-esteem has two parts: self-worth and self-efficacy. "Self-worth describes the degree to which a person "feels good" about him- or herself, and self-efficacy describes the sense that a person has that he or she can effect change, that his or her individual actions can have an impact on other people, policies, and/or institutions... Self-efficacy involves the empowerment and enablement of young people to actively do something about the world they live in, however modest the activity might be" (Scales 431). Community service may be just the means for achieving this end!

In the Search Institute's study of nearly 47,000 young and older adolescents prosocial behavior is identified as building social cohesion, functioning as a teacher, and reducing risky choices (*The Troubled Journey* 34). When asked, "During the last 12 months, how many times have you spent helping people who are poor, hungry, sick, or unable to care for themselves?" 40% of the 6th graders polled report none and 56% of the 10th-12th graders report none (36). Sixty-five percent of all those polled reported no weekly involvement in any form of volunteer work; non-helping seems to increase as grade in school increases (37).

Youth ministry and pastoral care emphasize the value of Christian service and discipleship, as modeled in Jesus' life and ministry. Yet we still struggle with mandatory vs. voluntary service opportunities, and service "projects" rather than service as a way of life. "Caring *is* an expression of the whole life and purpose of the Christian community" (Switzer 12). In the activity of caring, adolescents not only give but they receive, gaining insight into their own attitudes and abilities in the process. Therefore, prosocial opportunities are an integral part of who we are as church and what we are about. Every school and parish should pursue a wide variety of opportunities for young people to make a difference. Service activities should be encouraged throughout Confirmation preparation and the Christian Initiation process for both sponsors and candidates. Pairing young people with senior citizens who require individual assistance is a great opportunity for intergenerational sharing. "The combined approach of mentoring, peer helping, and community service may also represent a successful model of developing capable young people by increasing both their self-efficacy and their connection with others" (Scales 432). Teens are invaluable assets to a community as they serve others: as peer ministers, on community hotlines, as tutors in literacy programs and supervisors in latch-key programs, in shelters with homeless families, in child care centers, etc. Because service has such a powerful impact, it is given high school credit and considered a requirement in many states for graduation. Service helps create a sense of purpose, critical thinking, and support systems that we can't begin to reproduce through other programs and activities.

As youth ministers, we must examine the scope and the depth of our present service opportunities. Families must be encouraged to be involved in service together. It is much more than giving young people-something to do — it is allowing them to influence the world they live in, to provide opportunities for them to take leadership and ownership, to create change and learn to face the systems which surround them. In short, it's called building the kingdom of God — beatitude living.

MENTORING

To be effective, mentors must be persistent and resourceful. They must find ways to build trust that fit the particular individual and the cultural context in which they are working. They should know how to set tangible, usually modest goals early in the relationships. Mentors should be reasonably predictable and certainly dependable... They must know how to empathize with a developing adolescent, to be reasonably sensitive to what is current and choice, what is likely to be credible, and how to make sense out of the adolescent experience (Hamburg, 269).

If you think back on your own journey to adulthood, names and faces of significant adults will certainly come to mind. For me, there was a special teacher my junior year in high school, my pastor, a colleague at school, a resident assistant in college — all of whom were role models who influenced my choices of teaching, youth ministry, and counseling. "We must insure that our programs in youth ministry facilitate and nurture, rather than impede such relationships" (Dykstra 87). We have barely touched the tip of the iceberg in terms of effective mentoring relationships in youth ministry. Many of us have become too overworked and overprogrammed to pursue strong mentoring models and study the results. Yet the significance of mentoring is the individuality of the relationship.

Mentors are advocates, encouragers, resources, listeners, role models, guides, and companions. Presently, we operate on an adult relating to a group model (youth group, religious education class, sports team, leadership team, etc.) It has proven effective and efficient, but not very intimate. We are beginning to experiment but it is new turf, and we are very wary. We've begun with "Adopt-a-Grandparent" programs, spiritual directors for those older adolescents desiring a faith companion, retreat leaders, apprenticeships and internships. Mentoring might prove an exceptional process for those of you who have very few juniors and seniors involved in programs. It would provide an alternative format twice a month (mentors and mentees meet individually); once a month all juniors and seniors and their mentors gather; occasionally they join the entire group. It opens the door for exciting possibilities for them to be prepared to mentor another young person in the future.

Mentoring requires planning and visioning, but complements other pastoral care strategies. Of course, there needs to be training for these adults and young adults who are potential mentors. Once this is in place, it only need be refined each year. Presently, in my own diocese, mentors are a key component in our Lay Ministry Formation Program. Participants and mentors meet monthly, and mentors commit to a two year involvement. The continuity and the integrity of this relationship only serves to enhance the formation aspect of the program. Similar possibilities exist in youth ministry — adult prayer partners, mentors for justice and service activities, as Confirmation sponsors, for youth on parish councils and other committees. "The adolescent comes to feel a sense of personal worthiness just from seeing his or her particular and unique worth reflected in the eyes of an adult who is not a parent... Mentor relationships are not meant to last. But their impact is powerful. They provide a path through adolescence and a door into adulthood. They are never forgotten" (Dykstra 87, 89).

PARENT EDUCATION

Like every other aspect of youth ministry, pastoral care must extend beyond the framework of our ministry to and with youth, to include their parents and families. Adolescence challenges parents to understand, adjust, adapt, and respond to a variety of new situations and even crises. In trying to respond to their adolescent, many parents don't recognize the difference between disturbing and disturbed behaviors. Yet they truly want to do what is best for their developing adolescent. We, as youth ministers, often criticize parents for not being appropriately interested or involved in their child's faith formation. This is often one more expectation being placed on them in this increasingly demanding world. Many parents are overworked and overcommitted, trying to provide some quality time for their family. Many are struggling to meet the needs of their own aging parents. Whatever support and education we can offer to parents as they strive to achieve their own sense of identity, balance, and direction may prove to be a welcome relief. They are often just as overwhelmed as their teenagers with the pace of social change, yet are trying to help their children cope with issues they have never experienced.

The Church has just as much of a responsibility to work with parents as their children. It begins with helping them understand the adolescent's developmental needs and the needs of the family at their stage of the life cycle. Then we can begin to provide them with some of the faith foundations their children are learning, so they can be a resource and a support in family faith sharing as well as a sounding board for questions and criticisms. There could be parallel religious education opportunities for parents on the same faith themes their children are exploring, so that parents and teens can dialogue together. Parents need to be alerted to at-risk behaviors and warning signals so they know what is potentially harmful to their child's well being and what is "typical" adolescent behavior that will pass. Activities must be developed that families can participate in at-home: rituals, prayer experiences, videos, discussions, books, fun. Not everything needs to happen at the parish and, indeed, there should be one evening a week where nothing is scheduled at the parish — a Sabbath time where families can enjoy being together without running in six different directions. Parent support groups need to be encouraged, so parents know they're not in this alone. And even some informal parent gatherings where parents can socialize and youth ministry leaders can come to appreciate the richness of the families within the parish.

Pastoral care means we're all in this process together, and parents have often been neglected in this process. Newsletters, resource or media centers, access to counselors and other community experts, retreats, marriage enrichment, adult education, intergenerational programs, parenting classes, gathered and non-gathered opportunities should be made available to aid parents in developing confidence and competence to see their children through the teenage years.

> For the majority of our children, parenting is performed by one inexperienced biological relative; for the minority, it is performed by two inexperienced biological relatives who work full time and parent part-time... Nowadays, fewer people with fewer opportunities struggle to get this job done. Simultaneously, parenting faces more challenges than ever before in the form of drugs, drinking, sex, and dangerous, or at least ambivalent, messages from the media (Glenn and Nelson 47).

As a Church, it's time we encourage parents in this role and even join them in their role. Pastoral care is everyone's ministry.

PRAYER, RITUAL, SACRAMENTS

One of the most obvious, and least utilized pastoral care strategies are the ones we know and do best — prayer, ritual, and sacraments. Many young people have been alienated and hurt by the very ministers (and the institution) that call themselves "pastoral." Others see their parents refusing the sacraments and wonder why they should be a priority for them. We believe that there is an intrinsic connection between sacramental celebration and Christian living. How can we more effectively express this connection for adolescents and their parents and the entire faith community?

For me, it begins with the sacrament of Reconciliation, which is fundamentally a process of reincorporation into the Body of Christ. There should be flexibility in these rites to meet a variety of needs and expectations, as well as rich, symbolic action. We have not begun to tap into the power of healing, reconciling, sustaining, and comforting available in and through this sacrament. We need to provide on-going opportunities for reconciliation experienced beyond the regularly scheduled individual confessions — family celebrations, parish celebrations, catechesis for the sacrament with adolescents and their parents — and be creative, inclusive, and pastoral in our approach. These should occur at least seasonally, if not more frequently. However, the sacramental forms found in the Rite of Penance cannot bear the weight of the entire reconciliation process. We must also examine the pastoral possibilities which exist in the Eucharist — prayers of the faithful, involving families in presenting the gifts, involving adolescents in planning and ministry roles, the use of the homily, etc. There are also a variety of prayer and ritual experiences which call us to examine our experience as community — Liturgy of the Hours, Stations of the Cross, service to the local community, fasting, retreats, parish mission — and emphasize the need for conversion and outreach to the marginalized. Are there any rituals we have created and adopted as individual parish communities that celebrate our shared story? Do we model (or send home) rituals for Advent and Lent in particular that have a family focus? How does your parish celebrate World Youth Day ritually and liturgically? These are all statements of who we are and who or what we believe in and must be examined critically from time to time. How are people called to remember and pray for each other through phone chains, prayer groups, bulletins, announcements at Mass. Are those in need of prayer "inscribed" somewhere as a visible reminder?

This all adds up to a whole dimension of our pastoral life that is often neglected. If we are to actively take a stand in ways described earlier in this chapter, we must first of all be a prayerful community in every aspect. Pastoral care does not have to be complicated or extraordinary. It simply means taking advantage of ordinary opportunities to respond to people where they are, on *their* holy ground. Explore all the sacramental moments of your community life — they will reflect lived experience crying out to be recognized. Recognize it. Celebrate it.

SUMMARY

These are a few of the more promising pastoral care strategies. The important thing now is to take that first step. Select or create a strategy that will begin to move us to action. We must do more than simply be aware of the situation, we must actively work to change it.

What does it take now for children to grow up healthy and vigorous, inquiring and problem-solving, decent and constructive? In the years of growth and development, they need attachment, protection, guidance, stimulation, nurturance, and ways of coping with adversity. How can such experiences be provided? By an intact, cohesive family to the extent possible; by supportive, extended family and other social networks (Hamburg 331).

As Church, we play a critical role in determining the quality of life that children and adolescents have available. We must provide a vision of hope and a perception of opportunity by ministering the way Jesus did — affirming them, spending time with them, challenging the values of systems and society — through availability, vulnerability, compassion, and integrity, and the refusal to do it alone. "We can address such great problems effectively; we can relieve terrible suffering; we can stem the grievous loss of talent and life — if we have the vision and decency to invest responsibly in tomorrow's (and today's!) children and thereby in the future of all humanity" (Hamburg 333). It starts by moving out of the doorway — one step at a time!

Works Cited

Covey, Stephen R. *The 7 Habits of Highly Effective People.* New York: Simon and Schuster, 1989.

Dykstra, Craig. "Agenda for Youth Ministry: Problems, Questions, Strategies." *Readings and Resources in Youth Ministry.* Michael Warren, Ed. Winona, MN: St. Mary's Press, 1987.

Glenn, H. Stephen and Jane Nelson. *Raising Self-Reliant Children in a Self-Indulgent World.* California: Prime Publishing, 1989.

Hamburg, Beatrix, M.D. *Life Skills Training: Preventive Interventions for Young Adolescents.* Life Skills Training Working Group, Carnegie Council on Adolescent Development, 1990. (2400 N. Street, Washington, D.C. 20037, (202) 429-7979)

Hamburg, David A. *Today's Children.* New York: Random House, 1992.

Scales, Peter. "Developing Capable Young People: An Alternative Strategy for Prevention Programs." *Journal of Early Adolescence.* Vol. 10, No. 4, November, 1990.

Schorr, L. Within Our Reach: Breaking the Cycle of Disadvantage. New York: Doubleday, 1988.

Switzer, David K. *Pastoral Care Emergencies.* New York: Paulist Press, 1989.

CHAPTER 11

WHEN AND HOW TO REFER

David Switzer

OUR LIMITATIONS

Persons differ in their ability to help other persons in quandary and distress. Some rather obviously have higher levels of competence with a larger percentage of people with a greater variety of personalities, problems, and modes of relating. Even so, there are *no* Superhelpers (lay, clergy, psychotherapeutic professionals) who can be effective with all persons.

After all, we have different personalities ourselves, and there are simply some people who aren't going to "resonate" with us. There are those whom we're not going to like at all. There are those whose issues are going to stimulate anxiety in us, and our own defenses are going to click into place to protect us, which means, in some sense, protect us from intimacy in relationship with this particular person. None of us have been thoroughly educated and trained to understand and function with perfection with all kinds of persons and situations. Furthermore, our *feelings* of love and our commitment to help are simply not going to be sufficient to overcome these barriers. Case made? I hope so.

Ironically, I still discover some number of clergy (and therefore I would assume that there would also be some lay church professionals and volunteer church visitors) who believe that they can handle everything, that because they *care* (feeling) so much, just *love* (feeling) the person(s), and because they are so convinced of the power of faith, that all troubled people will have their problems resolved in interaction with them and with God. My impression is that the number of such clergy and lay care-givers is decreasing rather rapidly under the impact of their increased awareness of their own human limitations and the reality of the deep and persistent needs and complex behavior patterns on the part of some persons and family units.

My point is that we're only human, regardless of how self-aware and how well trained we are. Therefore, it's no sign that we're failures if, after talking with a troubled person a little while, we need to suggest that even though we can and will stay in touch, she or he really needs to be talking with someone else about this particular disturbing area of her or his life. With numerous people, it's the only responsible action that we can take. If we truly care, that is, are willing to *act* for the well-being of the other, the proper caring act is to help that person with this particular issue at this particular time be in touch with someone more competent and/or more available than ourselves.

There simply are, and always will be, some people that we cannot work with effectively *as the primary helper* in regard to their *psychological* problems. We may remain a primary helper with regard to issues of their faith, their spiritual development, and the behaviors which are expressions of faith. We may continue to be pastoral guides as other professionals work with them on the more complex psychological and interpersonal issues.

In regard to emotional and relational problems people have, we all have limitations as helpers. But let me point out some of the dimensions of limitations. In terms of the interaction between my competence and time and the nature of the other person and her or his particular problem, our limits have usually been portrayed as a *warning*:

There are critical human needs to which clergy and other representatives of the community of faith can effectively respond, using our own

LIMITS

CAREGIVER --------------------

Don't go beyond
this point.

This is accurate. It's critical. But it's not the whole story. It's equally important to recognize that there's a certain space within that boundary mark.

LIMITS

CAREGIVER --------------------

We can effectively
go this far.

genuine humanity, sensitivity, faith, and commitment to caring; carrying the power of being a living symbol of the Church, the faith, of God; and utilizing what knowledge and skills we do have.

The crucial issue, then, is that each one of us be able to make a relatively accurate assessment of our *own* limitations, recognizing that we clergy differ from other professional groups, individually we differ from one another, and all of us have different limitations at different times in our lives. We also differ from one another in terms of our levels of competence with different types of people and in different types of situations.

This relatively accurate assessment is no easy task. At times we may be very clear that we can or cannot be a primary caregiver to a person or family. Many other times we simply are not sure. There are at least two responsible courses of action when we are in doubt. First, we may consult with some appropriate professional person ourselves if that is possible. The process would be for us to review with the professional the characteristics and behaviors and history of the person we are working with, what we have done and haven't done thus far with the person, and our own feelings toward the person and within the helping relationship. This procedure, by the way, is not technically a violation of confidentiality. More important always than secrecy is the well-being of the person.

We're seeking consultation with the well-being of the troubled person(s) as the primary motivation, and we're doing it with a competent professional who herself or himself is now committed to the same confidentiality as we are with regard to the person(s).

Second, if such a professional person is not available to us, the most useful procedure is to refer the person to the professional, agency, or institution which has the highest probability of meeting the person's needs most adequately. Such a move also has some likelihood of avoiding possible dangers for that person and also for ourselves.

To review and systematize. Our limitations are defined:

1. By who we are as persons.

Apart from our pastoral care and counseling skills and a knowledge of procedures of intervention in different types of circumstances, some of us, because of our *emotional reaction*, can work with alcoholic persons and other drug abusers and some can't. Likewise some of us can and some of us cannot work with homosexual persons, with child or spouse abusers, with sexual voyeurs and exhibitionists, etc. Our own feelings can and do interfere with our establishing an adequate working relationship with persons with certain categories of problems. We need to be aware of this, candid with ourselves, and be willing and capable of making the most useful referrals or transferrals.

2. By our training and our experience.

Most clergy, lay church professionals, and other members of a congregation are not prepared to do long-term counseling of *any* kind, family therapy, to be the primary helping person for the severely emotionally disturbed, or for those whose critical problems are of long standing.

3. By our time.

Most clergy are generalists. We prepare and lead worship, preach, and minister the sacraments, oversee programs of Christian education and teach in several congregational settings, are responsible for the financial affairs of the congregation, direct other aspects of church programming, prepare personas for marriage and conduct weddings, represent the community in many community organizations and activities, call on the sick and dying and bereaved, lead the worship at funerals, and probably do a number of other things. Lay church professionals usually have their areas of specialty which are not pastoral care and counseling, and they are quite busy with these responsibilities. Volunteer lay caregivers very often have their own careers which call for a significant outlay of time and energy. We usually don't have time for anything but intervention in situational crises, one or two problem-solving, decision-making conversations, helping people in a marriage or a family become aware of a need for clearer and more open communication, short hospital and home visits, or limited assignments such as following one person through a long hospitalization or one family through their period of grieving.

At this point it is necessary to introduce the word "transferral." In this case, as well as when a person is homicidal, or psychotic, deeply depressed, in a situational crisis where other resources are desperately needed, we're responsible for helping that person get to the professional person(s), agencies, hospital, either by taking him or her ourselves, or, preferably, enlisting family members and/or other friends to assist. This action on our part is what may properly be called *transferral* instead of referral. In such instances, we're not merely making recommendations and seeking to elicit the others' cooperation in *their* taking the initiative to follow through on whatever action is appropriate. In transferral, we continue to work actively with and for a person with primary responsibility until she or he is in personal contact with the professional or agency or hospital which then assumes such responsibility (Switzer 1986, 102-04; Slaikeu 1984, 91-93).

No one of us can do it all. We all need each other, and we all need the psychotherapeutic, medial, social work, and other helping professionals. Therefore, let's take a look at when to refer, how to refer, and to whom to refer.

WHEN TO REFER

There are a number of ways of going about listing and discussing the circumstances under which it is either important or imperative that we make a referral or transferral of someone whom we're involved with as pastoral representatives of the Church.

The first and most obvious statement is that we do so any time we recognize that we're close to or beyond our own limits as these were portrayed in a general manner in the previous section.

There can be any number of more specific statements which can be guidelines for such actions, however. Such a list can never been entirely complete, because other persons with experience in caring can always think of yet another instance, and most of the ones which I shall list can usually be broken down into even greater detail. Several of them also overlap with one another. Many of the guidelines that follow are self-evident, and we can very easily be consciously aware of them. Others involve our own unconscious needs and conflicts. Therefore our perception of our strengths and weaknesses and our perceptions of the personality of the other and the meaning of that person's behavior can be hidden from us. It takes considerable perceptiveness on our part even to be aware of the clues given by certain distressed persons or by our own feelings and behaviors. Even when we become aware that there is probable cause to refer someone, we often feel our own resistance to such actions arising, and we want to keep on trying with this person.

With all of this said, here are a number of guidelines. We would be wise to refer when:

1. We simply don't understand what's going on with the other person, why the person feels and behaves as she or he does, even after we've had opportunity to talk with that person about what's going on.

2. We recognize that the person is psychotic or has a tenacious depression.

3. The person is suicidal or is making serious threats against someone else.

4. We suspect that the person may have some physical disorder, may need a physical examination, and/or may need medication.

5. A person is dependent on alcohol or some other chemical substance, including prescription drugs.

6. It had seemed as if this were a person appropriate to work with, but after a while we realize that no change is taking place, we're beginning to feel frustrated and we don't know what else to do.

7. We begin to be anxious too frequently with the person, consciously anxious or feeling ourselves usually being uptight.

8. We find ourselves beginning to shut the person out emotionally.

9. We feel consciously afraid because the person appears to be dangerous to us.

10. We feel angry at the person and aren't clear as to the reason.

11. We are sexually attracted to the person to the degree that our attention to him or her as a distressed human being is consistently (or very frequently) disrupted and our disciplined helping responses (the facilitative conditions) are compromised.

12. We want to take care of everything for the person and are not really helping the person to begin to be responsible for himself or herself.

13. We want to guard our relationship with the person and not let anyone else participate in significant helping with her or him.

14. The situation is primarily a family problem and the family pattern of interaction is complex.

15. We begin to see that, even if over a period of time we may be qualified to help, to do so effectively with this person or this family or in this type of situation means too much of our time and energy in the light of our other also important responsibilities.

In the section entitled, "By Our Time," I used the word "psychotic." This word refers to a variety of forms and intensities of loss of contact with reality and a severe disruption of a person's pattern of thinking and behaving which characterize severe mental illness. Most of the time these behaviors can be quite obvious as we observe a person or listen to the person talk about his or her experiences. There may be obvious delusions, usually of *extreme* suspicion, persecution, grandiosity, or references to the person's body: the woman speaking to me in the church office who said she was Queen Elizabeth; the man who looked me right in the eye as he told me of being so completely under the power of the devil that if the devil told him to kill me he wouldn't hesitate a second; the man in a hospital told me that he was dead and didn't have a body any longer. These are obvious! Delusions, of course, may be more subtle than these, but can usually be identified in conversation with someone.

All psychotic persons do not have hallucinations, but hallucinations comprise one of the symptoms of some number of people who are psychotic. The word "hallucination" refers to seeing, hearing, smelling, feeling insects or animals crawling on one, none of which is apparent to anyone else. It does need to be noted, however, that occasionally persons may have one or a few hallucinations without being psychotic (for example, as one behavior within a transient stage of normal grief).

Other significant changes in a person's behavior may indicate psychosis: fairly extreme withdrawal, not speaking at all, an uncharacteristic hyperactivity and inability to sleep normally, saying outrageous things that are out of characters with the person prior to this time, a breakdown of the person's usual rational thinking process, a loss of control leading to one impulsive act after another, talking without the usual reasonably logical connections between thoughts or with what the person has just finished saying, or with what someone else has just said, a flood of words almost without ceasing and rarely finishing sentences before going on to other ideas. An observant reader might recognize that most of us do some of these occasionally during temporary periods of distress. But what is being referred to as psychotic is a change in one's pattern of behavior which doesn't seem to be accessible to change by one's own thinking processes or by rational persuasion by another. The psychotic person usually is not able to critique his or her ideas and behaviors in the way he or she might formerly have done or the way in which most people do most of the time. Everyone who works with people in distress with any degree of frequency would do well to read a book on the sources and symptoms and treatment of mental illness.

Another disorder is clinical or psychiatric depression. Depression doesn't refer to having the blues for a couple of days or feeling down today or feeling sad for a longer period of time because of some loss. Unless covered up by other behaviors not always easily identified as being associated with depression, it is characterized by:

1. A rapid increase or decrease in appetite or weight.

2. Excessive or insufficient sleep.

3. Low energy level, tiredness, easily fatigued.

4. Psychomotor agitation and/or retardation.

5. Loss of interest and pleasure in usual activities.

6. Feelings of self-reproach and extreme guilt.

7. Decreased ability to think or concentrate.

8. Recurrent thoughts of death or suicide.

If a person has five or more of these particular symptoms, we may reasonably assume that the person is depressed (Rush). Other symptoms to look for are the appearance of sadness and the person's reporting of feeling sad, a sense of helplessness about doing anything about one's condition or situation, a sense of hopelessness about the future. Beck emphasizes that the *predominant* characteristic of psychiatric depression is a sense of hopelessness (1973, 21-22). He speaks of it in terms of "negative expectations." A depressed person may or may not also be truly psychotic. If psychotic, delusions are common, and also usually accompany the manic episode of bipolar depression (formerly called manic-depressive psychosis).

We need also always to keep in mind that certain moods and feelings and behaviors which are dysfunctional to a person, which are unpleasant and frightening to them, and which may often be disturbing or even dangerous to others, which seem to include symptoms of psychosis and/or depression, may not be of psychological origin, or entirely so. They may sometimes be the result of some psychological condition. So if a person's behavior has begun to change in significant ways, it is *always* imperative that the person see a physician.

Finally, we need to remember that some people can be dangerous, not only to themselves, but to others, including us. I truly believed the man who told me that if the devil were to tell him to kill me, he would. In his condition, he was capable of it. After our conversation, this man remained outside of the office with a family member while his son and I talked. I then called a psychiatric hospital and arranged an admission interview for the next morning. A family member stayed awake with him all night long, and the next day he was hospitalized.

In another tragic incident, a young man entered the office of a large metropolitan church. He asked to see a particular minister. That minister was not in that afternoon. The man went down the hall, found another minister, forced him into an office, and shot and killed him. The young man had a history of psychiatric difficulties, had been in a psychiatric hospital previously, had been attending a young adult group at the church, and the minister for whom he had asked the day of the killing had been "counseling" with him on and off for a fairly long period of time. The young man's behavior that had resulted from his fixation on the minister for whom he had asked was, to say the least, unusual and somewhat unrealistic and, for many people, would have been frightening.

My point certainly is *not* that all psychotic people are dangerous. They are not. Only a *very* small percentage are (somewhat like non-psychotic people). But there are behaviors which we need to pay attention to, and we cannot allow ourselves to believe that we can be primary counselors to them. We can, and should, of course, be pastors and friends, with a type of caution which is appropriate under certain conditions. A major way in which this caution is exhibited is in our doing all that we possibly can to see that such a person is under immediate psychiatric care.

HOW TO REFER

Barriers to Referral

There are at least three realistic barriers to referral.

The first is when we are living in a rural area or very small town where there are very few, if any, other psychotherapeutic professionals who live right in our area. Referral becomes somewhat more difficult, though seldom impossible, especially for the elderly and the poor. Questions to be raised are:

• How great is the person(s') need? Can we contribute something significant to the person(s) or can we not?

• If necessary, how skillful are we in helping the person(s) to see the degree of the need, and make some sacrifice themselves to go to the person or place where there is the greatest likelihood of the need being met?

• Are we willing ourselves to make the effort necessary to assist in the referral/transferral process?

I remember in my first parish a poverty stricken, illiterate, elderly couple. The wife desperately needed a type of operation that could be done in only a few hospitals in the state (and done free in only two or three). I made arrangements by phone through the chaplain's office in one of the hospitals located three and a half hours driving time from our rural area. These arrangements were both for the surgery and hospitalization as well as for a place for the husband to stay without cost. I drove them to the hospital, helped her get settled in the hospital and him into his room, and drove back, about twelve hours for the entire trip, little enough investment for the seriousness and urgency of the need. Arrangements were made for someone else to bring them home a week or ten days later. It was all possible and it was worth it.

Counseling and psychiatric care, other than hospitalization, is often difficult to locate. But even in these cases, there are beginning to be counselors in smaller towns, mental health centers in larger towns, and psychiatrists, clinical and counseling psychologists, and psychiatric social workers in very small cities. The highways are usually good, and many people are already accustomed to driving thirty minutes to a couple of hours for things of lesser importance. For the poor and elderly, we can organize car pools.

The second, somewhat more formidable barrier to referral, is when we ourselves really don't want to do it. This resistance may be conscious or unconscious on our part. Either way, we truly believe that *we* are the *one* person the other needs, even though we are somewhat aware that one or more of the criteria for referral mentioned above are present. To put it crassly, we're saying, "I'm this person's (this family's) only hope." This is usually a delusion of somewhat grandiose proportions, and it's very rarely true. When we find ourselves beginning to feel this way, it's usually a sign that referral is *definitely* called for. We then need to find our own counselor and talk about this reaction of ours. (You had better believe that I've done this myself, although unfortunately I waited rather late in my career to begin. The psychiatrist's question to me has always been in words more or less like the following: "What need of *yours* is so strong that it was being met in a relationship where *you* were supposed to be working to see that the *other* person's needs were being attended to?" From there, we got down to the specifics.)

A third obstacle in referral is when the other person doesn't want to talk with anyone else: for examination, evaluation, or counseling. This often thrusts us back to dealing with obstacle number two, as the person tells us how much we've meant to him or her, what wonderful people and helpers we are, how understanding. They don't want to have to start all over with someone else. Often, they say they won't. We begin to feel forced into the position of beginning to think that if the person doesn't work with me, she or he won't be in touch with anyone else, so — once again, "I'm the person's only hope." We must be as rigorously honest as we can be *with ourselves first*, and then with the other person. How do we assess the person, her or his situation, and our ability to help? Can we recognize that we simply *are not* capable of assisting the type of change that needs to take place in the person's or family's life, or do we even have serious doubts about it? In these instances, we don't contribute to the person(s) involved by continuing to be the only or primary caregiver. We must then explain to the person or persons that our genuine concern for their well-being leads us to recommend that they see someone else who will really be able to help them more effectively than we can. We emphasize, if it be the case, that we shall continue to be their friend, their pastor, and that we shall stay in contact and support them. If the person or persons refuse the referral, we need to be firm in our commitment to them as friend, lay minister, or pastor, but also be clear that we can't and won't be the only one or primary one they call upon for the resolution of critical life problems.

The Process of Referring

Some people initially respond to the suggestion that they talk with someone else rather than us with the feeling of being rejected, believing that we don't want to talk with them anymore, and/or that they must be worse off than they had thought they were.

Therefore, the process of referring takes time and sensitivity and skill. It's not something we do in the last couple of minutes of a conversation, snapping off, "Oh, by the way, you need to talk with Dr. Edmonds. Here's his phone number," or "It sounds as if you need to make an appointment at Family Guidance rather than talking with me about this situation."

Clinebell (316-20) and Oglesby (Ch. 3) give very helpful and detailed guidelines for the referral process. As soon as we begin to recognize that referral or transferral may be necessary, we begin to respond in ways that might help the person(s) grasp that even though we seem to understand them and their situation, we're not the most competent person to assist with this type of problem or issue they are presenting to us. This involves our communication both of how we perceive what they are describing and our own particular limitations. We work with them to help them clarify their own understanding of their situation and how it is that we are not really the best facilitator of its resolution. We then indicate that there are others who are specially trained and who have experience in the particular area and discuss how these persons (or agencies or institutions) function to assist in a condition or situation like theirs. If we ourselves have any doubt as to whether the person needs to be referred, or if we don't know where to suggest that the person might go, we need to seek consultation ourselves from a specialist who can help us with our decision and with the process.

We express our caring for the person or persons that we are seeking to refer and assure them that for them to see someone else doesn't mean that we have stopped caring or that we no longer will have pastoral conversations with them. Then at some point, we ask them how they would feel about seeing the particular professional or going to a certain agency. A few people will now respond immediately or fairly quickly that it's something that makes sense to them and they will do it. They're grateful for the type of help that we have given them.

Others, of course, and usually for understandable reasons, will express their resistance or reluctance. We spend time with them, assisting them in expressing any feelings of rejection and hurt they have toward us, any irritation, their anxiety about themselves or about beginning over again with someone whom they don't know. This stage of the procedure cannot be rushed. If there condition or situation allows it, we might even have another conversation with them a day or two later. We need to be careful that our own anxiety doesn't lead us to abbreviate this discussion or that the others' resistance in whatever form (anger or emotional seduction) doesn't trigger our fear or our need to be needed and lead us to renege on our recommendation of referral.

Many people will complete the process by taking the next helpful step, going to the appropriate referral source. We reassure the persons of our continued concern. We arrange follow-up steps with them by asking them to give us a call or stop by after the first appointment with someone else, or, if hospitalized, assure them that we will visit.

Some people will either say that they will go to the person or place referred and not do so. Others will make it clear that they don't intend to do so. If they can't talk with us, they're not going to talk with anyone. That is their decision. We have done what we could in their best interests, and they have refused to take these steps for themselves.

Where To Refer

Nothing is more helpful than a referral to a person, agency, institution, program, or the appropriate combination of these where a person or family realizes that here is the place and person(s) who know how to work with them in a way that some or many of their important needs are probably going to be met.

Few things are more frustrating for needy persons than to have been talking to someone and have this person whom they've known or gotten to know refer them on to someone else or some other place which they then discover is *not* the appropriate place to be. So they must then go on to someone else. This process only tends to increase the frustration of persons who are already anxious and distressed, probably angering them, leaving many of them with additional resistance to any other referral.

A significant part of competent referring is to know well, and as much as possible personally, as many as possible of the resources of one's own geographical area: different types of professionals and their areas of specialty and/or greatest competence; what certain agencies do and do not do and what they cost; various programs, their location and meeting times, who operates them, who is eligible for them, whether there are fees, and, if so, how much they are; what hospitals specialize in what types of disorders; the details of commitment proceedings to psychiatric hospitals, etc.

The second major part of making the referral is getting to know sufficiently well the relevant details of a particular person's or family's condition and situation so that the person or family and the referral resources can be matched with confidence.

Since relatively few people know everything, we may sometimes not be certain as to the proper referral. Therefore, with any given person or family, we may have to do additional research. I've often picked up the phone while the person or persons I've been talking with are still there to make from one to three calls gathering information so that the best match may be made between them and one or more resources.

Certainly every clergy and lay pastoral caregiver needs to realize that all physicians are not psychiatrists and are not necessarily fully up-to-date on medication such as anti-depressants and tranquillizers, that psychiatrists *are* physicians and that many very competent psychiatrists don't do group therapy or family therapy; that psychiatric social workers cannot hospitalize persons as psychiatrists can do, but often are the very ones to do group or family therapy; that all social workers are not therapists; that clinical psychologists are specialists in evaluation and usually do individual therapy in a competent manner, but that they may or may not do family therapy, cannot prescribe medication, nor in most states directly hospitalize persons, although in a few states they are permitted to do so, that all psychologists are not clinical or counseling psychologists and therefore do other sorts of things entirely.

It is probably appropriate for many lay visitors to check with the ordained clergy of the congregation concerning the referral of the person the lay caregiver has been visiting. For example, the lay visitor might not have known how to handle a particular situation or question that has arisen in discussion with someone in the hospital or with the family in grief. He or she may merely consult with the clergy as to how to respond more effectively to the sick or bereaved. Sometimes it may be useful for the ordained pastor to make a visit to the person or family in question. The layperson may discover other referrals with the person he or she has been visiting. Perhaps it would be important for the sick or bereaved or the distressed person to have a conversation with the most competent person on the staff in the pastoral care in order to see whether or not the staff member might become the primary helper or whether a referral needs to be made. Occasionally the minister may become the primary crisis counselor when the lay person is untrained in that area.

All of this is said in the realization that in a number of congregations there are members who know more about some aspects of these matters than do the clergy, so a layperson may recommend a particular physician or counselor or agency, or the ordained minister may often consult with members of the congregation who themselves are in the helping professions or who know about agencies and programs which the clergy person is not aware of.

There may be times when a distressed person or family does require the particular services that can be offered by a psychiatrist or clinical or counseling psychologist, but yet the nature of the problem is such that they would need a counselor with the time and specialized training beyond that of most clergy in local congregations. At the same time, there may be very good reasons for the person(s) to be working intensively with a counselor who is well educated in the various theological disciplines or even who is ordained. Parish clergy need to be aware that in many locations there are pastoral counseling centers where such specialists are performing their ministry. They are in almost every large city, many small cities, and increasingly in larger and a few smaller towns. They are usually, though not always, interdenominational. No one would really expect them all to be of the same quality, so the responsible clergy or lay person would want to check on their work before making a referral, just as we would do with any other professional.

It's obvious that appropriate referring is a team effort. When this takes place within the congregation, the designated ordained clergy (the only one, the senior one, the one assigned to this area) is usually the coordinator of the team. The coordinator is one who knows many but not all of the referral resources and who continually draws upon the knowledge of members of the parish.

Two of the most important things any clergyperson can do upon coming to a new parish is

(1) to find out what persons in the congregation are members of the helping professions, whether they are in independent practice or related to an agency, institution, or program; get to know them personally and then use their expertise in whatever ways are helpful in the total caring program of the church; and (2) to discover as many as possible of the other resources; get to know personally as many helping professionals as she or he can; visit agencies; make appointments with directors of programs,

halfway houses, etc. Concentrating this activity in the early weeks and months of one's ministry in a new parish will pay tremendous dividends in the longer-term future. These dividends will not be confined only to the pastoral caring activities of the minister and the congregation. There will be in addition an increase of understanding and good will on the part of an increasing number of professionals and the agencies and programs which they represent.

Works Cited

Beck, Aaron L. *The Diagnosis and Management of Depression.* Philadelphia: University of Pennsylvania Press, 1973.

Clinebell, Howard. *"Referral Counseling." Basic Types of Pastoral Care and Counseling.* (Revised and enlarged) Nashville: Abingdon Press, 1984.

Oglesby, William. *Referral in Pastoral Counseling.* Nashville: Abingdon Press, 1978.

Rush, M.D., John. Lecture given at the University of Texas Southwestern Medical School. Dallas, Texas.

Slaikeu, Karl A. *Crisis Intervention: A Handbook for Practice and Research.* Boston: Allyn and Bacon, 1984.

Switzer, David K. *The Minister as Crisis Counselor.* (Revised and enlarged) Nashville: Abingdon Press, 1986.

CHAPTER 12

PLANNING AN INTEGRATED APPROACH TO PASTORAL CARE

Sharon Reed

This country and its people have a great capacity to respond to crises and to launch large-scale interventions to rescue the victims of disasters. The time for hand-wringing about the status of youth has passed and now communities, with support from the states and the nation, have to get down to the hard work of creating a viable system for the future (Dryfoos 269).

We too, as Church, must move beyond questioning what has happened to our young people and how it will impact "the-church-of-the-future." That slogan has done us a disservice. It has allowed us to adopt a "why face today if we can put it off until tomorrow" mentality. Now we can no longer afford to "put off" young people. We have the information needed to provide a broad spectrum of responses to the systems, situations, and risks they encounter. This begins by making pastoral care a priority in all our parishes. We cannot be content with simply *naming* pastoral care as important. We *must* move beyond naming the response to *action*.

As we have seen in this book, pastoral care includes strategies for *prevention* — promoting healthy adolescent development, strategies for *caring* with youth in crisis — responding to youth in need, and strategies for *advocacy*. Using this broad, more inclusive understanding of pastoral care we now turn our attention to creating an integrated approach to pastoral care in our parish or school settings. This chapter will propose an approach to pastoral care that is collaborative, pro-active, decisive, and far-reaching. It will involve each of us in examining how our parishes, families, schools, and communities educate, support, nurture, challenge, encourage, and equip young people to deal with the world in which they live.

We will examine how to use four major approaches to planning an integrated approach to pastoral care: [1]

1) Integrating pastoral care attitudes, strategies, and activities into existing youth programming;

2) Incorporating a family perspective into pastoral care strategies and activities;

3) Utilizing and/or collaborating with community programs/resources (parish ministries/programs, agencies/organizations and resources in the civic community, diocese, state or country);

4) Designing new pastoral care programs or services.

APPROACH 1

Integrating Pastoral Care into Existing Youth Programming

In Chapter 8, I outlined an approach that integrated pastoral care into each of the components of youth ministry as outlined in *A Vision of Youth Ministry*: word (evangelization and catechesis), worship, community life, guidance and healing, justice and service, enablement/leadership development, and advocacy. While guidance and healing may be the component that is primarily focused on pastoral care, the entire *Vision* statement is an endorsement and validation of the necessity for pastoral care in each of the seven components. In order to reenergize and revitalize our current approach to promoting positive adolescent development, we must integrate pastoral care into all that we are about, as well as address the implications of a ministry rooted in pastoral care principles and perspectives. This will include strategies for *prevention, caring,* and *advocacy.*

Using pastoral care as a lens, we can view many of the programs, services, and ministries of a parish or school community as opportunities for prevention, caring, and advocacy. This will involve a process of reflection and analysis. We ask ourselves how we can integrate a pastoral care perspective into everything we are doing. What are the current pastoral care programs/ministries and resources in the faith community? What opportunities are already available for restructuring? It might be as simple as introducing several pastoral care themes into a catechetical program or designing a parent component to accompany a catechetical course or program. It might include redesigning a retreat experience. In my diocese we offered a second-level leadership training called "You Can Make a Difference" and integrated a service day in the middle of the training. The service activity was experienced, processed, and critically analyzed in light of leadership principles and its ability to create change. It was the one component participants continually asked to have repeated. It might mean contacting a counselor or organization in the community to run a support group on a recovery topic, such as substance abuse, divorce, etc. The possibilities are as varied as our ministries and the needs of youth and families.

Integrating a pastoral care response into existing programming involves being aware of what is already happening and how it can be enhanced by introducing a new activity, by using new program resources, or by networking with parish or community leaders and resources. It encourages us to *look for opportunities* for pastoral care and to bring them to the attention of others.

Potential Strategies for Integrating Pastoral Care

Here is a listing of strategies we have already proposed in this book: (See Chapters 2, 8, and 10 for further descriptions of each of these strategies.)

• Promote positive values in all programming.

• Develop social competence and social skills — life skills training.

• Create networks and social supports for youth and families.

• Create opportunities for youth to be contributing members of the Church community.

• Provide caring and supportive relationships in the Church community and youth programs.

• Create mentoring relationships, programs, and systems.

• Partner with parents and families.

• Provide parent education, encouragement, support networks, and resources.

• Provide a variety of meaningful, stimulating, challenging and constructive youth activities and programs. Provide catechesis for Christian living.

• Provide meaningful service involvements for young people.

• Utilize the power of healing, reconciling, sustaining, and comforting found in the sacraments, in prayer, and in ritual.

• Engage youth in leadership and leadership training.

• Address specific at-risk concerns among youth with information and connect these concerns to Christian faith and values.

• Uphold high expectations for adolescents.

• Get involved in community networking, cooperation and collaboration to address the needs of young people.

APPROACH 2

Incorporating a Family Perspective intoProgramming

How are the services and ministries of the youth program made available to families? This may sound like an absurd question, but when we focus most of our energy on serving individuals and/or building community among teens in the youth ministry, the question is worth asking because families often become fragmented in the process... The youth ministry program can help create an atmosphere of support for families that helps them prioritize activities, say "no" to some of society's demands, and rediscover the value of home life. When the minister emphasizes quality home life, it will surely enrich the ministry as well (Kehrwald).

We've heard about family perspective for years; doing it successfully is quite a different thing. A family perspective in youth ministry means looking at our ministry and programs through a "family lens," and making appropriate adjustments. It means doing all we can for youth and their families without always creating new programs. Pope John Paul II in his Exhortation on the Family, *Familiaris Consortio*, captured the essence of family perspective when he wrote, "No plan of organized pastoral work at any level must ever fail to take into consideration the pastoral area of the family." In particular it means:

a. Viewing individuals in the context of their family relationships and other social relationships. As a systems orientation, a family perspective is a lens that focuses on the interaction between individuals, their families, and social institutions (*Family Perspective* 8).

b. Using family relationships as a criterion to assess the impact of the Church's and society's policies, programs, ministries, and services. As a criterion to assess ministry, a family perspective provides a means to examine and adjust systematically policies, program design, and service delivery. Its goal is to incorporate a sensitivity to families and to promote the partnership, strengths, and resources of participating families (*Family Perspective* 8).

A family perspective in ministry with youth seeks to:

• Sensitize the minister to the realities of marriage and family life.

• Sensitize those who serve individuals to broaden their perspective by viewing the individual through the prism of adolescent household life.

• Helps adolescent families become better partners with the many institutions they deal with regularly...including the parish itself (Kehrwald).

Effective pastoral care means helping young people and their families successfully negotiate the changes of adolescence, including the spiritual and moral challenges. We must work hard to help parents and families see youth ministry and the faith community as a resource for them. We will have to be sensitive to the unique demands of our partnership with families. We will have to provide a variety of pastoral care programs and services for the diversity of family structures in our communities — two-parent, single parent, blended or step-families, adoptive families, and dual career parents. Unless we really know our audience, our programs and pastoral care approaches will be ineffective.

Creating a family perspective in pastoral care can take many forms. Four comprehensive strategies can guide our thinking:

1. Incorporating a family perspective and family involvement into current program. This involves examining our current pastoral care efforts and bringing family concerns into youth programming, connecting with the realities of family life, applying the learnings from a youth program into family life, and/or involving families (or parents) in pastoral care programming with their teens.

2. Creating in-home resources and activities. Helping families grow in faith and build stronger relationships is the goal of in-home resources and activities. This can take a variety of forms such as providing parenting resources (print or video), family rituals and celebrations, (e.g., a family reconciliation service), and family activity suggestions. Many current youth and adult programs can be redesigned to include a take-home resource or activity for the family. Newsletters can become an excellent vehicle for communicating in-home activities and parenting suggestions.

3. Resource center. Giving parents and family members access to quality print, video, and community resources is the goal of a resource center. A resource center becomes an information clearinghouse and rental library for families and leaders. The center would contain resources (books, videos, pamphlets) on parenting, improving family relationships, family activities, community resources (counseling services), etc.

4. Provide parent education, encouragement, support networks, and resources. Many current research studies point to the need for building the competence and confidence of parents through parent education training and resources. Parishes can provide an important service to parents and the community by placing a priority on providing organized, systematic parent education, and by intentionally creating support groups and networks for parents.

Potential Strategies for Incorporating a Family Perspective into Pastoral Care Programming

Here are ideas for translating the four comprehensive strategies into action.

- Meet youth on their "home turf"
- Be involved with parents
- Parent advisory group
- Parallel needs assessment for parents
- Bridging experiences
- Reentry experiences
- Family life awareness raisers
- Parent education programs
- Programs for parents and adolescents
- Parent component of a youth program
- Parallel programs for parents
- Parent/family resource center
- Newsletters
- Home-based resources

APPROACH 3

Utilizing and Collaborating with Existing Programs and Resources

Many parishes continue to invest time, energy, and money on programs that are being done or could be done by other sectors of the community. Using a pastoral ministry perspective means that we do not reinvent the wheel; instead, we wisely use the pastoral care resources (organizations, people, print and audio-visual) that are already present in our areas. Churches need to work with other community organizations in a common effort to promote healthy adolescent development. Sharing resources, co-sponsoring programming, mobilizing the community to address youth issues are only some of the ways churches and community organizations can work together for the common good of all young people.

In order to initiate this approach to pastoral care, a parish or school will need to investigate what is currently happening in the community and what resources already exist. Every parish and school should have a directory of community resources and programs. This directory should include the offerings of other churches and synagogues, social service agencies, youth organizations, schools, libraries, counseling services. Each entry in the directory should list the agency, contact people, programs sponsored and services offered, schedules, materials available, etc. Since many parishes connect with multiple middle schools and high schools, this research would provide a valuable picture of the structures and supports offered by various school systems. It would also alert us to parishioners who are teachers, social workers, counselors, youth professionals, or who have access to valuable programs or resources. How could they be involved more intentionally in pastoral care efforts?

One idea for using your directory of community resources is to develop and distribute a list of recommended adolescent and family counseling resources with their services and fees that youth and their families can use for assistance in times of trouble. Youth ministers should meet some of them personally, discuss methods of referral, values, and how they could collaborate to provide family counseling to those who need it. A parish or school can print cards with phone numbers of crisis intervention services, support groups, resource people and agencies. The directory can also include a list of community educational programs and resources (books and videos) for youth and/or parents that address adolescent/family concerns and problems.

A second idea is to create a calendar that lists all of the *recommended* parish and community events for youth and for families in a given month or season (3-4 months). This is a great way to alert youth and their families to upcoming programs, activities, and events and to invite them to participate. Make sure that the calendar includes pertinent information on each event. Mail the calendar to every youth and their parents or insert it into the parish bulletin. Be sure to highlight parish activities. This calendar could also list school vacations, musicals, parent programs, dates newsletters are published, as well as policies, support groups offered, special events, retreats, and needs as far as volunteers or specific parish support.

Our research should surface what programs are sponsored by other churches in your area and what speakers are available from the diocese and other community sources? In my area, we have wonderful speakers sponsored by the YMCA/YWCA, area hospitals and churches, and special interest groups. Sometimes it's helpful to have check the local papers each month, send for area church bulletins, and get on mailing lists of pertinent groups so that the parish youth ministry can publish monthly pastoral care programs.

Our research should also uncover opportunities to work with other concerned leaders and organizations to lobby politicians on youth and family issues.

Collaborating with other organizations and leaders means that we don't need to organize everything alone. We can use the time and talent of youth and adults in our parish or school to help us focus on what is already happening in the community. We *do* need to know what's already happening and creating a positive impact. This will go a long way toward alleviating overlap.

Recommendations for Community Leaders from the Search Institute

• Assemble a permanent child and youth task force involving leaders from all community sectors. Ideally, raise funding to permanently staff the task force.

• Create a community-wide vision for positive youth development.

• Continually assess progress toward the vision through systematic exploration of youth perceptions, behavior, values and needs.

• Create a detailed action plan to promote positive youth development with an emphasis on increasing youth access to effective schools, families and youth-serving organizations.

• Advocate for greater state or federal support for school effectiveness, parent education, day care and after school care, prevention programming, and other efforts crucial for promoting positive youth development.

• Ensure that one's community offers a range of support services for families and structured, adult-led activities for youth (*The Troubled Journey*).

APPROACH 4

Designing New Pastoral Care Programming

Once we are aware of how pastoral care perspectives can be infused into already existing programming and have seen the value of collaboration on a broad-based level, the next step is to identify the gaps or unmet needs and design the necessary programs to fill them. (Even designing new programs can be done collaborating with other churches or community agencies concerned about the issue.) New programming arises because of our desire to respond to the unmet needs of youth in our particular environment.

The challenge in new programming is to reach the targeted young people and their families using the best possible resources and prevention/intervention strategies available. Youth ministry has prided itself on its ability to combine personal presence with powerful programming. Now however, we are dealing with young people who are at risk in multiple areas, possess fewer social supports, and lack many of the necessary life skills. "One in four children of the 28 million aged 10 to 17 are in dire need of assistance because they are at high-risk of engaging in multiple program behaviors — of being substance abusers, having early unprotected intercourse, being delinquents, and failing in school" (Dryfoos 245). Much of our present programming is not prepared to respond adequately to this dilemma. We need to be more pro-active in advocating for funding to sustain specialized programs, in working with other leaders and organizations in our communities, and in encouraging more creative programming led by peers.

PLANNING FOR PASTORAL CARE

The *Pastoral Care Activity Manual* contains a detailed Planning Guide which is designed to assist you in creating pastoral care opportunities in your particular setting, using the four approaches described in this essay. It is meant to be both simple and flexible, so adapt the process and the forms to meet the needs of your community. Hopefully, it will provide the foundation for integrating pastoral care into all aspects of youth ministry.

End Notes

[1] Much of the outline used in this section are adaptations of Chapter 7, "Organizing Parent Education" by John Roberto in *Faith and Families*, edited by Thomas Bright and John Roberto (New Rochelle: Don Bosco Multimedia, 1992).

Works Cited

Benson, Dr. Peter L. *The Troubled Journey: The Profile of American Youth.* Minneapolis, MN: RespecTeen, 1990.

Bright, Thomas and John Roberto, editors. *Faith and Families.* New Rochelle, NY: Don Bosco Multimedia, 1992.

Curran, Dolores. *Working With Parents.* Circle Pines, MN: American Guidance Service, 1989.

Dryfoos, Joy G. *Adolescents at Risk.* New York: Oxford University Press, 1990.

Hamburg, David A. *Today's Children.* New York: Random House, 1992.

Kehrwald, Leif and John Roberto, editors. *Families and Youth — A Resource Manual.* New Rochelle, NY: Don Bosco Multimedia, 1992.

A P P E N D I X

RESOURCES FOR PASTORAL CARE

PASTORAL CARE: FOUNDATIONS

Aleshire, Daniel O. Faithcare: *Ministering to All God's People Through the Ages of Life*. Philadelphia: Westminster Press, 1988.

Arnold, William V. *Introduction to Pastoral Care*. Philadelphia: Westminster Press, 1982.

Augsburger, David W. *Pastoral Counseling Across Cultures*. Philadelphia: Westminster Press, 1986.

Borchert, Gerald L., and Andrew D. Lester, eds. *Spiritual Dimensions of Pastoral Care: Witness to the Ministry of Wayne E. Oates*. Philadelphia: Westminster Press, 1985.

Capps, Donald. *Pastoral Care*. Philadelphia: Westminster Press, 1979.

Clinebell, Howard. *Basic Types of Pastoral Care and Counseling*. Nashville: Abingdon Press, 1984.

Duffy, Regis. *Roman Catholic Theology of Pastoral Care*. Philadelphia, Fortress Press, 1983.

Hart, Thomas. *The Art of Christian Listening*. New York: Paulist Press, 1980.

Kennedy, Eugene. *Crisis Counseling*. New York: Continuum, 1981.

Kennedy, Eugene and Sarah Charles, M.D. *On Becoming A Counselor* (Expanded Edition). New York: Continuum, 1991.

Mayeroff, Milton. *On Caring*. New York: Harper & Row, 1971.

Switzer, David K. *The Minister as a Crisis Counselor*. Nashville: Abingdon Press, 1974.

Wicks, Robert J. *Availability: The Problem and the Gift*. New York: Paulist Press, 1986.

Wicks, Robert J. *Self-Ministry Through Self-Understanding*. Chicago: Loyola University Press, 1990.

Wicks, Robert J. *Seeking Perspective: Weaving Spirituality and Psychology in Search of Clarity*. New York: Paulist Press, 1991.

Wicks, Robert J., Richard Parsons, and Donald Capps, editors. *Clinical Handbook of Pastoral Counseling — Volume 1* (Expanded Edition). New York: Paulist Press, 1993.

Wicks, Robert J. and Richard Parsons, editors. *Clinical Handbook of Pastoral Counseling — Volume 2*. New York: Paulist Press, 1993.

PASTORAL CARE: SKILLS

Bolton, Robert. *People Skills*. New York: Simon and Schuster, 1979.

Covey, Stephen R. *Principle Centered Leadership*. New York: Summit Books, 1991.

Covey, Stephen R. *The 7 Habits of Highly Effective People*. New York: Summit Books, 1988.

Egan, Gerard. *The Skilled Helper*. Monterey: Brooks/Cole, 1975.

Faber, Adele and Elaine Mazlish. *How To Talk So Kids Will Listen and Listen So Kids Will Talk*. New York: Avon Books, 1990.

Ferris C.S.J., Margaret. *Compassioning — Basic Counseling Skills for Christian Care-Givers*. Kansas City, MO: Sheed & Ward, 1993.

Kramer, Patricia. *The Dynamics of Relationships: A Guide for Developing Self-Esteem and Social Skills*. (Equal Partners. 11348 Connecticut Ave., Kensington, MD 20895 (301-933-1489)

Moore, Joseph. *Helping Skills for the Nonprofessional Counselor*. Cincinnati: St. Anthony Messenger Press, 1992.

Vaughan, Richard P. *Basic Skills for Christian Counselors*. New York: Paulist Press, 1987.

PASTORAL CARE: ADOLESCENTS

A Matter of Time. Carnegie Council on Adolescent Development. New York: Carnegie Corporation of New York, 1993.

Barnes, Jr., Robert G. *Confident Kids*. Wheaton, Ill.: Tyndale House Publishers, 1987.

Benson, Dr. Peter L. *The Troubled Journey: The Profile of American Youth*. Minneapolis, MN: RespecTeen, 1990. (Call 1-800-888-3820 for a free copy of the study.)

Dryfoos, Joy G. *Adolescents at Risk*. New York: Oxford University Press, 1990.

Elkind, David. *All Grown Up and No Place to Go*. New York: Addison-Wesley Publishing, 1984.

Fields, Doug. *Too Old Too Soon*. Oregon: Harvest House, 1987.

Glenn, H. Stephen, and Jane Nelson. *Raising Self-Reliant Children in a Self-Indulgent World: Seven Building Blocks for Developing Capable Young People*. Rocklin, CA: Prima Publishing & Communications, 1988.

Hamburg, David. *Today's Children — Creating a Future for a Generation in Crisis*. New York: Times Books, 1992.

Hewlett, Sylvia Ann. *When the Bough Breaks — The Cost of Neglecting our Children*. New York: Basic Books, 1991.

Ianni, Francis. "A Structure for Adolescent Development." *Access Guides to Youth Ministry: Early Adolescent Ministry*. Ed. John Roberto. New Rochelle, NY: Don Bosco Multimedia, 1991.

Ianni, Frances. *Search for Structure*. New York: Basic Books, 1989.

Lester, Andrew D. *When Children Suffer*. Philadelphia: Westminster Press, 1987.

Lester, Andrew D. *Pastoral Care with Children in Crisis*. Philadelphia: Westminster Press, 1985.

Kehrwald, Leif and John Roberto, editors. *Families and Youth — A Resource Manual*. New Rochelle, NY: Don Bosco Multimedia, 1992.

Louv, Richard. *Childhood's Future*. New York: Doubleday, 1991.

Parsons, Richard D. *Adolescents in Turmoil, Parents Under Stress: A Pastoral Ministry Primer*. New York: Paulist Press, 1987.

Roberto, John, editor. *Access Guides to Youth Ministry: Early Adolescent Ministry*. New Rochelle, NY: Don Bosco Multimedia, 1991.

Rowatt, G. Wade. *Pastoral Care with Adolescents in Crisis*. Louisville: Westminster/John Knox Press, 1989.

Scales, Peter C. *A Portrait of Young Adolescents in the 1990s*. Carrboro, NC: Center for Early Adolescence, 1992.

Shelton, Charles. *Adolescent Spirituality*. Chicago: Crossroad Publishing, 1983.

The State of America's Children 1992. Children's Defense Fund. Washington, DC: CDF, 1992.

Steinberg, Lawrence and Ann Levine. *You & Your Adolescent*. New York: Harper Perennial, 1990.

Van Ornum, William and John Mordock. *Crisis Counseling With Children and Adolescents*. New York: Continuum, 1990.

Van Pelt, Rich. *Intensive Care: Helping Teenagers in Crisis*. Michigan: Youth Specialties, 1988.

PASTORAL CARE: FAMILIES

Allen, Mary Lee, Patricia Brown, and Belva Finlay. *Helping Children by Strengthening Families*. Washington, DC: Children's Defense Fund, 1992.

Ackerman, Norman J. *A Theory of Family Systems*. New York: Gardener Press, 1984.

Ambrose, Dub and Walt Mueller. *Ministry to Families with Teenagers*. Loveland, CO: Group Books, 1988.

Curran, Dolores. *Working with Parents*. Circle Pines, MN: American Guidance Service, 1989.

Curran, Dolores. *Traits of the Healthy Family*. San Francisco: Harper & Row and New York: Ballatine Books, 1983.

Drey, Janet. *Families and Young Adolescents*. New Rochelle, NY: Don Bosco Multimedia, 1992.

Guarendi, Ray. *Back to the Family: How to Encourage Traditional Values in Complicated Times*. New York: Villard Books, 1990.

Guernsey, D. *A New Design for Family Ministry*. Elgin, IL: David Cook Publisher Co., 1982.

Kehrwald, Leif and John Roberto, editors. *Families and Youth — A Resource Manual*. New Rochelle, NY: Don Bosco Multimedia, 1992.

Larson, Jim. *A Church Guide for Strengthening Families*. Minneapolis: Augsburg, 1986.

NCCB. *A Family Perspective in Church and Society*. Washington, DC: USCC, 1988.

NCCB. *Putting Children and Families First*. Washington, DC: USCC Publishing, 1991.

NCCB. *A Catholic Campaign for Children and Families Parish Resource Manual*. Washington, DC: USCC Publishing, 1991.

Power, Thomas A. *Family Matters — A Layman's Guide to Family Functioning*. Meredith, NH: Hathaway Press, 1989.

Roberto, John, editor. *Growing in Faith: A Catholic Families Sourcebook*. New Rochelle: Don Bosco Multimedia, 1990.

Ross, Richard and G. Wade Rowatt, Jr. *Ministry with Youth and Their Parents*. Nashville: Convention Press, 1986.

Small, Stephen. *Preventive Programs that Support Families with Young Adolescents*. New York: Carnegie Corporation of New York, 1990.

The State of America's Children 1992. Children's Defense Fund. Washington, DC: CDF, 1992.

Steinberg, Laurence, and Ann Levine. *You and Your Adolescent — A Parent's Guide for Ages 10-20*. New York: Harper & Row, 1990.

Stinnett, Nick and John DeFrain. *Secrets of Strong Families*. Boston: Little, Brown, and Co., 1985.

Strommen, Merton and Irene. *Five Cries of Parents*. San Francisco: Harper and Row, 1985.

PASTORAL CARE: SPECIAL ISSUES

Apthorp, Stephen P. *Alcohol and Substance Abuse*. Wilton, CT: Morehouse-Barlow Co., 1985.

Barun, Ken and Philip Bashe. *How to Keep the Children You Love Off Drugs*. New York: The Atlantic Monthly Press, 1988.

Bauman, Ph.D., Lawrence with Robert Riche. *The Nine Most Troublesome Teenage Problems And How to Solve Them*. New York: Ballantine Books, 1986.

Blackburn, Bill. *Caring in Times of Family Crisis*. Nashville: Convention Press, 1987.

Emmett, Steven Willey, ed. *Theory and Treatment of Anorexia Nervosa and Bulimia*. New York: Brunner/Mazel, 1985.

Comstock Herbruck, Christine. *Breaking the Cycle of Child Abuse*. Minneapolis: Winston Press, 1979.

Cottman Becnel, Barbara. *Parents Who Help Their Children Overcome Drugs*. Los Angeles: Lowell House, 1989.

Cretcher, Dorothy. *Steering Clear*. Minneapolis: Winston Press, 1982.

Crook, Marion. *Teenagers Talk About Suicide*. Toronto: NC Press Limited, 1988.

Doyle, Patricia and David Behrens. *The Child in Crisis*. New York: McGraw-Hill Book Company, 1986.

Ellis, Dan C. *Growing Up Stoned*. Pompano Beach, FL: Health Communications, Inc., 1986.

Feindler, Eva L., and Randolph B. Ecton. *Adolescent Anger Control*. Elmsford, NY: Pergamon Press, 1986.

Husain, Syed Arshad. *Suicide in Children and Adolescents*. Jamaica, NY: Spectrum

Publications, 1984.

Shelp, Earl E., and Ronald H. Sunderland. *AIDS and the Church*. Philadelphia: Westminster Press, 1987.

Eschner, Kathleen Hamilton, and Nancy G. Nelson. *Drugs, God & Me*. Loveland, CO: Group Books, 1988.

Giffin, M.D., Mary and Carol Felsenthal. *A Cry for Help*. Garden City, NY: Doubleday & Company, Inc., 1983.

Joan, Polly. *Preventing Teenage Suicide*. New York: Human Sciences Press, Inc., 1986.

Kageler, Len. *Helping Your Teenager Cope with Peer Pressure*. Loveland, CO: Group Books, 1989.

Klaus, Tom. *Healing the Hidden Wounds*. Loveland, CO: Group Books, 1989.

Marshall, Shelly. *Young, Sober & Free*. New York: Harper/Hazelden, 1978.

McCoy, Kathleen. *Coping with Teenage Depression — A Parents' Guide*. New York: New American Library, 1982.

McLenahan Wesson, Carolyn. *Teen Troubles — How to Keep Them From Becoming Tragedies*. New York: Walker Publishing Company, Inc., 1988.

Meehan, Bob with Stephen J. Meyer. *Beyond the Yellow Brick Road — Our Children and Drugs*. Chicago: Contemporary Books, Inc., 1984.

Perkins, William Mack and Nancy McMurtrie-Perkins. *Raising Drug-Free Kids in a Drug-filled World*. New York: Harper/Hazelden, 1986.

Polson, Beth and Miller Newton, Ph.D. *Not My Kid — A Parent's Guide to Kids and Drugs*. New York: Avon Books, 1984.

Sheppard, Kay. *Food Addiction, The Body Knows*. Pompano Beach, FL: Health Communications, 1987.

Williams, Dorthy and Lyle. *Helping Your Teenager Succeed in School*. Loveland, CO: Group Books, 1989.

Smith, Ph.D. Manuel J. *Yes, I Can Say No — A Parent's Guide to Assertiveness Training for Children*. New York: Arbor House, 1986.

Woititz, Janet G., *Adult Children of Alcoholics*. Pompano Beach, FL: Health Communications, 1983.

Youngs, Ph.D, Bettie B. *Helping Your Teenager Deal with Stress*. Los Angeles: Jeremy P. Tarcher, Inc., 1986.

PASTORAL CARE: SPECIFIC STRATEGIES

3:00-6:00 P.M. Programming

Dorman, Gayle. *3:00-6:00 P.M.: Planning Programs for Young Adolescents*. Carrboro: Center for Early Adolescence, 1985.

Lefstein, Leah, William Kerewski, Elliot A. Medrich, and Carol Frank. *3:00-6:00 P.M.: Young Adolescents at Home and in the Community*. Carrboro: Center for Early Adolescence, 1982.

Opportunities for Prevention: Building After-School and Summer Programs for Young Adolescents. Adolescent Pregnancy Prevention Clearinghouse. Washington, DC: Children's Defense Fund, 1987.

Life Skills Training

Glenn. H. Stephen. *Developing Capable People Leader's Package*: Leaders Manual, Six Cassette Tapes, Participant's Workbook. Provo, UT: Sunrise Associates, 1990. (Spanish version available)

Glenn, H. Stephen, and Jane Nelson. *Raising Self-Reliant Children in a Self-Indulgent World: Seven Building Blocks for Developing Capable Young People*. Rocklin, CA: Prima Publishing & Communications, 1988.

Hamburg, Beatrix. *Life Skills Training: Preventive Interventions for Young Adolescents*. New York: Carnegie Corporation of New York, 1990.

Hamburg, David. "Teaching Life Skills and Fostering Social Support." *Today's Children — Creating a Future for a Generation in Crisis*. New York: Times Books, 1992.

Advocacy

NCCB. *A Catholic Campaign for Children and Families Parish Resource Manual*. Washington, DC: USCC Publishing, 1991.

Welcome the Child. Children's Defense Fund. Washington, DC: CDF, 1991.

Mentoring

Flaxman, Erwin, Carol Ascher, and Charles Harrington. *Youth Mentoring: Programs and Practices*. New York: Institute for Urban and Minority Education. (212-678-3433)

National Mentoring Working Group. *Mentoring: Elements of Effective Practice*. Washington, DC: One to One. (202-338-3844)

Milestones in Mentoring: A Training Program for Volunteer Mentors. (Video series with guidelines) Pittsburgh, PA: One PLUS One. (412-622-1491.

Mosqueda, Patricia Flakus, and Robert Palaich. *Mentoring Young People Makes a Difference*. Denver: Education Commission of the States. (303-830-3692)

Saito, Rebecca and Eugene Roehlkepartain. "The Diversity of Mentoring." *SOURCE* 7.4 (November 1992). (Available through the Search Institute, 612-376-8955)

The Two of Us: A Handbook for Mentors. Baltimore: The Baltimore Mentoring Institute. (301-685-8316)

Vitek, John. *A Companion Way — Mentoring Youth in Searching Faith*. Winona, MN: St. Mary's Press, 1992.

Parenting Adolescents

Active Parenting: Teaching Cooperation, Courage, and Responsibility. Michael Popkin. Marietta, GA: Active Parenting, 1986.

Video: In addition to the video presentations the *Active Parent Handbook* and *Action Guide* help viewers understand and remember the information and skills shown by the 40 video segments. They contain review exercises, home activities and family enrichment suggestions. Sessions: I: *The Active Parent*, II: *Understanding Your Child*, III: *Instilling Courage*, IV: *Developing Responsibility*, V: *Winning Cooperation*, VI: *The Democratic Family In Action*. (2 hours each — 6 videos; EcuFilm)

Active Parenting in the Faith Community — A Biblical and Theological Guide. Freda Gardner and Carol Rose Ikeler. Atlanta: Presbyterian Publishing House.

Boys Town Videos for Parents. Distributor: Don Bosco Multimedia; Video 10-16 minutes each — 11 videos.

The *Boys Town Videos for Parents* series covers topics from self-esteem and peer pressure to making sure teens and preteens do their homework and help around the house. The tapes are packed with concise information and are lively and dramatic, with true-to-life vignettes that illustrate key points. A booklet with additional information accompanies each video. Titles: *A Change for the Better: Teaching Correct Behavior; Catch 'Em Being Good: Happier Kids, Happier Parents Through Effective Praise; Homework?: I'll Do It Later!; I Can't Decide: What Should I Do?; I'm Not Everybody: Helping Your Child Stand Up To Peer Pressure; It's Great to be Me!: Increasing Your Child's Self-Esteem; Negotiating Within the Family: You and Your Child Can Both Get What You Want; No I Won't And You Can't Make Me!; Setting Your Child Up for Success: Anticipating and Preventing Problems; Take Time to Be a Family: Holding Successful Family Meetings; You Want Me to Help with Housework? No Way!*

Bringing Families Together: Parent Education Programs. Lorraine Amendolara, Eileen Murphy and Mary Longo. Huntington, IN: Our Sunday Visitor, 1990.

Four Leader Books with parent handbooks: *Good Beginnings, Growing Up Together, Parents and Teens Together, Communicating Christian Sexuality to Children.* The fifth leader book, *Establishing Parish Parenting Centers*, is an organizing manual.

Creating Family Intimacy, Love and Sex. (Video Program) Distributor: Franciscan Communications; 50 minutes each — 5 videos.

A five part video program that helps parents understand family relationships, filmed before a live audience that weaves modern research with Clayton Barbeau's own professional experiences. Titles: *Husband/Wife Relationships, Creating Family, The Male/Female Crisis, Teens, Singles and Love Vs. Sex, Parents as Role Models*

Developing Capable People Leader's Package: Leaders Manual, Six Cassette Tapes, Participant's Workbook. H. Stephen Glenn. Provo, UT: Sunrise Associates, 1990. (Spanish version available)

Raising Self-Reliant Children in a Self-Indulgent World: Seven Building Blocks for Developing Capable Young People. H. Stephen Glenn and Jane Nelson. Rocklin, CA: Prima Publishing & Communications, 1988. (Parent Book)

Empowering Teenagers and Yourself in the Process. Jane Nelsen and Lynn Lott. Provo, UT: Sunrise Associates, 1990. (7-Tape Audio Program with Study Guide)

I'm On Your Side: Resolving Conflict with Your Teenage Son or Daughter. Jane Nelsen and Lynn Lott. Rocklin, CA: Prima Publishing & Communications, 1990. (Parent Book)

Faith and Families — A Parish Program for Parenting in Faith Growth. Thomas Bright and John Roberto, editors. New Rochelle, NY: Don Bosco Multimedia, 1992. (Organizers Manual)

Parenting for Faith Growth Series. New Rochelle, NY: Don Bosco Multimedia, 1992.

Parents of Adolescent books: *Families Experiencing Faith: A Parents' Guide to the Young Adolescent Years, Families Exploring Faith: A Parents' Guide to the Older Adolescent Years.*

Living with 10-15 Year Olds. Gayle Dorman, Dick Geldof, and Bill Scarborough. Carrboro, NC: Center for Early Adolescence, 1982.

Workshops on four topics: Living with 10-15 Year Olds, Parents and Young Adults: Talking About Sex, Risk-Taking Behavior and Young Adolescents; Understanding Early Adolescence.

214 Guides to Youth Ministry Series

Early Adolescence: What Parents Need to Know. Anita Farel. Carrboro, NC: Center for Early Adolescence, 1982. (Parent Book)

Parenting for Peace and Justice — Ten Years Later. Jim and Kathleen McGinnis. Maryknoll: Orbis Books, 1990.

Training Program: *Building Shalom Families: Christian Parenting for Peace and Justice.* Jim and Kathleen McGinnis. St. Louis, MO: *Institute for Peace and Justice,* 1986.

Complete video package containing: two 120-minute VHS videotapes, 32-page guidebook, Parenting for Peace and Justice book, and worksheets and action brochures.

Parenting: Growing Up Together Series. (Video Program) Distributed by: EcuFilm; 20-22 minutes each — 6 videos.

This six video program shows us not only how we can be better parents, but how in the process of parenting we can continue our own growth. Led by Laura Knox and Cynthia Candelaria, nationally-known parent counselors, authors and workshop leaders, the programs feature discussions and interviews with a diverse mix of parents, whose children span the full spectrum of ages from infant to adult. The accompanying leader's guide clearly outlines how the programs can be easily and effectively used as a series or individually, with either adults or youth. Titles: *Expectations, Feelings, Communicating, Exploring Problems, Solving Problems, Letting Go.*

Parenting Teenagers Set I: *What Makes Your Teenager Tick?; Parenting, How Do You Rate?; Communicating With Your Teenager; Your Teenager's Friends and Peer Pressure*

Parenting Teenagers Set II: *Effective Teenage Discipline; How to Talk About Sex and Dating; School: Helping Your Kids Measure Up; Building Christian Faith in Your Kids*

(Group Publishing; Each set: 30 minutes — 4 videos. Includes leader guides with helpful insights, publicity tips and ready-to-copy worksheets).

Practical Parenting. (Video) Distributor: Brown/Roa Media; 30 Minutes each — 6 videos.

This is a six-part video parenting program featuring the work of noted expert, Dr. Bill Wagonseller and narrated by actor Dick Van Patten. Study booklet included with each video. Titles: So You're Going to be a Parent, School Days, The Art of Communication, Child Management, Single Parenting, Adolescence.

Responsive Parenting. Saf Lerman. Circle Pines, MN: American Guidance Service, 1984.

Parent Packet (set of 9 booklets): *Helping Children as They Grow* — ages and stages, *Helping Children Help Themselves* — discipline, *Helping Siblings Get Along Together* — includes new baby, *Using Role Reversal with Children, Building a Child's Positive Self-Image, Sharing Sex Information with Children, Helping Children Handle Fear* — includes death, *Helping Children Understand and Express Feelings* — includes divorce and remarriage, *Building Independence and Cooperation in Children.*

Complete Kit: Leader's Manual, Participant's packet, 3 Audiocassettes, 10 Charts, and Publicity Aids.

STEP/teen: Systematic Training for Effective Parenting of Teens. Don Dinkmeyer and Gary D. McKay. Circle Pines. MN: American Guidance Service, 1990. (Parent Book)

STEP/teen Kit for the Trainer: Leader's Guide, Parent Handbook, 5 Audiocassettes or 2 Videocassettes — includes script booklet, STEP for Substance Abuse Prevention Booklet, and Publicity Packet.

STEP/teen Biblically. Rev. Michael Bortel. Circle Pines, MN: American Guidance Service, 1989. (Parent Book)

Leader's Manual: STEP/teen Biblically. Rev. Michael Bortel. Circle Pines, MN:

American Guidance Service, 1989.

Strengthening Your Stepfamily. Elizabeth Einstein and Linda Albert. Circle Pines, MN: American Guidance Service, 1986. (Parent Book)

Complete Kit: Leader's Guide, Participant's packet — includes parent book and Encouragement Packet with 30 at-home activities, 3 Audiocassettes, Wall Charts, Blackline Masters, and Publicity Aids.

Teaching Parenting. Jane Nelsen and Lynn Lott. Provo, UT: Sunrise Associates, 1988.

This parenting manual provides a step-by-step approach to starting and leading experientially-based parenting groups. *Teaching Parenting* is a program that can be used alone or with other parenting programs. The manual includes outlines for use with eight major parenting books, including *STEP, Active Parenting, Positive Discipline.*

Understanding Your Teenagers. Wayne Rice. LaJolla, CA: Youth Specialties, 1992.

A six-session video-based parenting program with facilitator guide.

Single Parent and Blended Family Resources

Barnes, Jr., Robert G. *Single Parenting.* Wheaton, IL: Tyndale House Publishers, 1987.

Bonkowski, Sara. *Kids are Nondivorceable: A Workbook for Divorced Parents and Their Children.* Chicago: ACTA Publications, 1990.

Bradley, Buff. *Where Do I Belong? A Kid's Guide to Stepfamilies.* Reading, MA: Addison-Wesley, 1982.

Einstein, Elizabeth. *The Stepfamily: Living, Loving and Learning.* New York: Macmillan Co., 1982

Einstein, Elizabeth, and Linda Albert. *Strengthening Your Stepfamily.* Circle Pines, MN: American Guidance Service, 1986.

Einstein, Elizabeth, and Linda Albert. *Stepfamily Living: Preparing for Remarriage.* Ithaca, NY: E. Einstein Enterprises, 1983.

Evans, Marla D. *This Is Me and My Two Families: An Awareness Scrapbook/Journal for Children Living in Stepfamilies.* New York: Brunner-Mazel.

Francke, Linda Bird. *Growing-Up Divorced: How to Help Your Child Cope with Every Stage —from Infancy through the Teens.* New York: Fawcett Crest, 1983.

Getzoff, Ann, and Carolyn McClenahan. *Stepkids: A Survival Guide for Teenagers in Stepfamilies.* New York: Walker and Co., 1984.

Ives, Sally B., David Fassler, and Michele Lash. *The Divorce Workbook: A Guide for Kids and Families.* Burlington, VT: Waterfront Books, 1985.

Lewis, Helen Coale. *All About Families the Second Time Around.* Atlanta: Peachtree Publishing, 1980.

Mayle, Peter. *Divorce Can Happen to the Nicest People.* New York: MacMillan, 1979.

Monkres, Peter R. *Ministry with the Divorced.* New York: Pilgrim Press, 1985.

Seuling, Barbara. *What Kind of Family Is This? A Book about Stepfamilies.* Racine, WI: Western Publishing, 1985.

Visher, Emily B. and John S. Visher. *Stepfamilies: Myths and Realities.* Secaucus, NJ: Citadel Press, 1979.

Service

Bright, Thomas and John Roberto, editors. *Access Guides to Youth Ministry: Justice.* New Rochelle: Don Bosco Multimedia, 1990.

Condon, Camy and James McGinnis. *Helping Kids Care: Harmony Building Activities for Home, Church and School*. St. Louis: Institute for Peace and Justice, 1988.

The Earth Works Group. *50 Simple Things You Can Do to Save the Earth. 50 Simple Things Kids Can Do to Save the Earth. The Next Step: 50 More Things You Can Do to Save the Earth*. Berkeley, CA: Earthworks Press.

Hollender, Jeffrey. *How to Make the World a Better Place*. New York: William Morrow and Co., Inc., 1990.

Lewis, Barbara A. *The Kid's Guide to Social Action*. Minneapolis: Free Spirit Publishing Inc., 1991.

MacEachern, Diane. *Save our Planet — 750 Everyday Ways You Can Help Clean Up the Earth*. New York: Dell Publishing, 1990.

McGinnis, James. *Journey into Compassion — A Spirituality for the Long Haul*. St. Louis: Institute for Peace and Justice, 1989.

McGinnis, James, ed. *Helping Teens Care*. New York: Crossroad Publishing Co., 1991.

Office on Global Education, Church World Service. *Making a World of Difference*. New York: Friendship Press, 1989.

Roehlkepartain, Eugene C. *Building Bridges: Teens in Community Service*. Minneapolis, MN: RespecTeen, 1991. (Call 1-800-888-3820 for a free copy.)

Salzman, Marian, and Teresa Reisgies. *150 Ways Teens Can Make Difference*. Princeton, NJ: Peterson's Guides, 1991.